the

portion teller

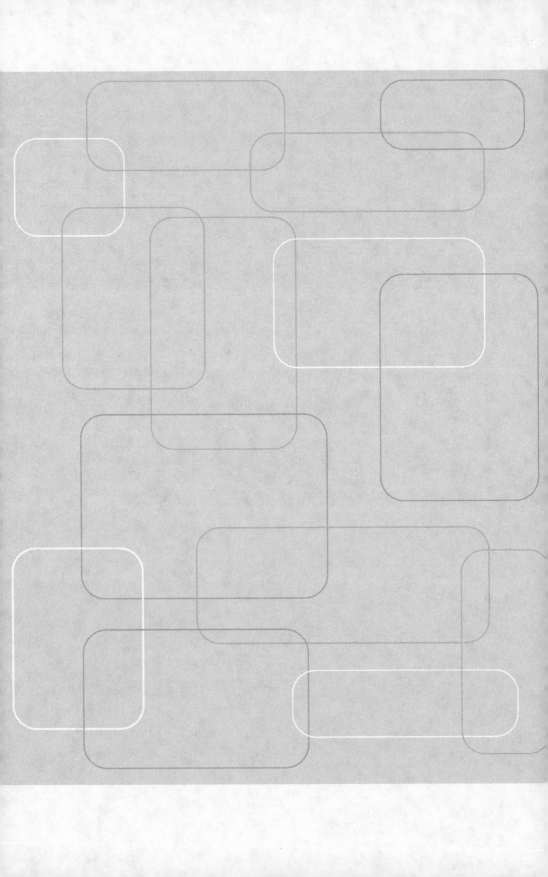

the

portion teller

smartsize your way

to permanent

weight loss

LISA R. YOUNG, PH.D., R.D.

Morgan Road Books
New York

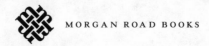

MORGAN ROAD BOOKS

Published by Morgan Road Books, an imprint of The Doubleday Broadway Publishing Group, a division of Random House, Inc.

Morgan Road Books and the M colophon are trademarks of Random House, Inc.

Disclaimer: This book is not intended to take the place of medical advice from a trained medical professional. Readers are advised to consult a physician or other qualified health professional regarding treatment of their medical problems. Neither the publisher nor the author takes any responsibility for any possible consequences from any treatment, action, or application of medicine, herb, or preparation to any person reading or following the information in this book.

PRINTED IN THE UNITED STATES OF AMERICA

Visit our Web site at www.morganroadbooks.com

First edition published 2005

Book design by S · C Design
Interior illustrations by Sydney Vandyke for Art Department

Library of Congress Cataloging-in-Publication Data
Young, Lisa R.
The portion teller : smartsize your way to permanent weight loss /
by Lisa R. Young.—1st ed.
p. cm.
Includes bibliographical references.
(alk. paper)
1. Weight loss. 2. Reducing diets. 3. Food portions. 4. Nutrition.
I. Title.
RM222.2.Y683 2005
613.2'5—dc22 2004062528

ISBN 0-7679-2068-6

1 3 5 7 9 10 8 6 4 2

In memory of my beloved grandparents

To my grandmother, Celia Aronson, for her strength and determination throughout her life, and for inspiring me and encouraging me to pursue a career in nutrition. And to my grandfather, Jessie Aronson, whose words of wisdom—follow it up, keep the door open, and always leave a sweet taste—remain with me forever. You both taught me to think big and start small.

acknowledgments

I would like to express my sincere appreciation to the following people who helped make this book a reality. *The Portion Teller* would not have been possible without the guidance and support of terrific colleagues, friends, and family.

I am so grateful to Marion Nestle, my mentor and thesis advisor at New York University (NYU), for her inspiration, guidance, and sincere interest in my work; and for her valuable time and generosity during all stages of this project. I am thankful to my agent, Lydia Wills, for believing in this book from the get-go, and for providing terrific advice, encouragement, and support throughout. A special thanks to Jason Yarn for keeping things running smoothly.

I felt warmly encouraged and supported by the publishing team at Morgan Road Books. I am grateful to my publisher, Amy Hertz, for her immediate enthusiasm for this project, her vision, expertise, and excellent suggestions; and to my editor, Marc Haeringer, for his commitment, terrific feedback, availability, and helpful advice. Much thanks to others at Morgan Road Books, including David Drake, Anne Watters, and Nate Brown.

I would like to express my appreciation to Adrienne Forman for reading the entire manuscript and offering thoughtful suggestions; and to Jodi Citrin, Carly Nemirow, Shoshana Werber, and Jessica Yep for excellent research assistance. And many thanks to my clients who brought real issues to the table and helped me to develop practical solutions.

I am very fortunate to have terrific colleagues and friends who provided helpful suggestions, assistance, and support throughout. My deepest gratitude to Robert Barnett, James Barron, Pamella Darby, Carol Durst, Jodi Eisen, Naftali Robert Friedman, Shona Goodman, Ari Goodman, Michele Harris, Emil Hedaya, Jamillah Hoy-Rosas, Heather Kouffman, Andrew Kramer, Hilary Liftin, Karen Miller, Eva Stein, and Sheldon Watts.

I am indebted to my dedicated dissertation committee at NYU for their support while conducting my academic research on portion sizes, which planted the seeds for this book. A special thanks again to Marion Nestle for being the most wonderful thesis advisor anyone could ever have, and to Jeffrey Backstrand and Sharon Weinberg for their helpful advice and encouragement. I would like to express my appreciation to the Department of Nutrition, Food Studies, and Public Health at NYU for awarding me a departmental scholarship and to Dean Patricia Carey for awarding me the Dean's Grants for Student Research award for the funding of this research. I am also grateful to the many nutrition professionals, food companies, and food personnel willing to speak with me and share their information.

Finally, my love and appreciation to my wonderful family for their love, support, and encouragement not just throughout this process but throughout my entire life. Words cannot express my gratitude. Thank you, Mom and Dad, Bonnie, Luca, Teo, Celia and Brando.

contents

foreword

I hardly know anyone who is not worried about gaining weight, here in the United States or just about anywhere else. This is not just a matter of how you look. The more overweight you are, the greater your chance of having diabetes (the adult-onset kind), high blood pressure, and high blood cholesterol, all of which can increase your chance of having a heart attack. You may be one of the lucky people who can gain weight and still be healthy, but most of us would be much better off eating less and being more active.

For normal mortals, eating less is not so easy. Perhaps for reasons of evolution, we are programmed from birth to eat as much as we can any chance we get, as if another good meal will never come again. We finish what is in front of us. The more in front of us, the more we eat. As Dr. Lisa Young explains so eloquently in this book, it's large portions that cause the problems. Larger portions have more calories. The more calories you eat, the more weight you can gain.

Lisa Young and *The Portion Teller* to the rescue! When Lisa was doing her doctoral degree with me at New York University, her terrific idea was to go out and measure the actual sizes of foods people were eating. Obvious as this might seem, nobody had done it. She discovered that the foods served now are enormous compared to what the government defines as a standard serving size. They also are enormous compared to what Americans ate thirty years ago. What she found will amaze you. As soon as food companies started making larger portions in the early 1980s, people ate more. When they ate more, their weights went up. By now, so many other researchers have confirmed her work that the remedy is clear. If you want to keep from gaining weight, you need to watch your portion sizes. *The Portion Teller* tells you how, and gives you a fresh approach to managing weight—one that makes perfect sense. If you are trying to lose weight, or just want to know how much you and your family are actually eating, Lisa Young's *The Portion Teller* is an invaluable resource. It's also great fun to read. Enjoy it and use it!

MARION NESTLE, PH.D., M.P.H.
Paulette Goddard Professor,
New York University

introduction

*I've been on a constant diet for the last
two decades. I've lost a total of 789 pounds.
By all accounts, I should be hanging from
a charm bracelet.*

● ERMA BOMBECK

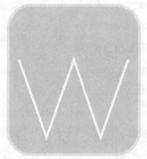hen I started counseling people on how to lose
weight in the late 1980s, I heard many diet war
stories. The same complaints came up over and
over again: The food is boring. I feel hungry. I feel
deprived. There are too many rules. The most
common lament was: How can I possibly follow
all these rules for the rest of my life? I saw firsthand that no matter how successful a strict diet is in the short term, it rarely works in the long run. At the
same time as I was learning these stories of dieting failures from my clients, I
started noticing something going on around me—the size of food was growing. I noted the extra mound of pasta at dinner, the increase in the diameter
of a pizza, the ballooning of bagels, the upward creep of all fast-food and
restaurant portions. This change was pretty gradual, so most people didn't
pay attention. It wasn't until recently, when the word "supersize" became part
of the vernacular, almost a cliché to describe overgrown portions, that people started to realize what was happening to their food—and to their bodies.

Along with the supersize culture came a supersize America that has collectively gained weight at an unprecedented rate in the past few decades.

As I gathered more information about the growth of portion sizes for my Ph.D. at New York University, I knew that any weight-loss program had to take into account two things: (1) a realistic, personalized eating plan that works for life, and (2) an education in exactly how large portions had become, retraining perceptions. Instead of seeing just another muffin, I wanted my clients to see a *huge* muffin. And then smartsize it!

I developed this program because I didn't think that the diets out there were realistic. Not only are they hard to follow, but they seem to ignore how large our foods have become. Look around you at the diet programs today—almost all of them are based on the idea that you have to cut certain foods, or even entire food groups, from your diet. They claim that it's the carbs, the fat, or the sugars that are making you fat. The entire diet industry seems to focus on what we put in our mouths rather than how much of it we consume. They focus on which foods are good or bad, healthy or unhealthy, a "diet" food or a restricted food. This approach is at odds with how people really eat. It's not the carbs or the fats that are making us gain weight. It's not *what* we eat, it's *how much* we eat. It's portion size that is making us fat.

Did you know that a typical bagel today has almost the same calories and nutrient value as five slices of bread? You probably wouldn't think twice about having a bagel on the run, but you would know you were overdoing it if you grabbed five slices of bread on the way to the office. Once you know what a bagel is "worth," you'll see your breakfast in a new way. You won't need calorie charts, weights, scales, or calculators to understand what a healthy portion is. There's no getting around it: In order to lose weight, you have to limit calories. But on this program, you won't have to count them! What you'll do is develop portion-size awareness. You'll get a basic understanding of what your body needs and *how much* of it you should be eating. Armed with this awareness, you can go anywhere—out to dinner, an all-you-can-eat buffet, a cocktail party, or a home-cooked meal—and know exactly how much you're eating. All you need to do is to smartsize instead of supersize.

With smartsizing, there are no rigid prescriptions, no "first week on, second week off" foods—in fact, no restricted foods whatsoever. It's all about awareness: portion-size awareness, nutrition awareness, and self-awareness. You can eat what you want as long as it fits into your own eating plan. The beauty of this program is that you can take it as far as you want; you can work the entire program, which includes detailed instructions on how to keep the Portion Teller Diary, tips and activities for downsizing your portions, and specific strategies for dining out, shopping, and making your home more portion-friendly. Or you can choose instead to focus on a basic understanding of portion sizes and put portion control into action in your daily life, leaving a few bites on your plate at a restaurant, eating only half a sandwich, or switching from a large glass of orange juice to a fresh orange. If you make these changes and no others, you can lose between ten to twenty pounds in one year without even feeling the pinch of deprivation. Small, simple changes add up. I've watched it happen with my clients countless times, and I know we can make smartsizing work for you.

Smartsizing doesn't promise a magic pill, instant weight loss, or overly dramatic results in the first few days. What it does offer is a time-tested, personalized, and sane alternative to unhealthy crash diets with short-term results. Smartsizing works. I've seen client after client—many who spent years on the up-and-down yo-yo diet-go-round—lose weight by smartsizing and keep it off for the long run, all the while eating foods they love. Nothing makes me happier than a client who says, "I never knew it was so easy. I don't stress out about food anymore." If you smartsize it, you won't have to change your life, just your relationship to food. By the end of the book, I guarantee that you will never look at an oversized restaurant entrée, a humongous muffin, or a mound of pasta the same way again. Instead, you will see your food in terms of healthy portions. Again, the choice of exactly how much and what you eat will be up to you. The Portion Teller program gives you everything you need to make your own choices, eat the foods that you love, and still lose weight and keep it off. Welcome to diet liberation.

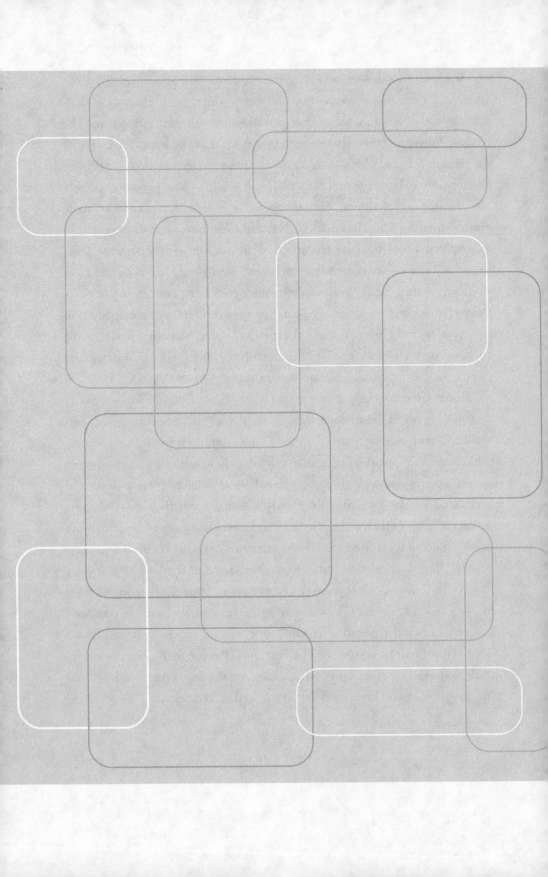

america expands

*I've been on a diet for two weeks
and all I lost is fourteen days.*
• TOTIE FIELDS

f you've said anything like this recently, you're not alone. We spend enormous amounts of time, energy, and money on weight-loss programs, diet pills, shakes, prepackaged low-cal meals, fat- and sugar-free foods, and the latest diet books and products that promise a quick fix for our weight problems. The sad fact is that our investments are not paying off. No matter what we seem to do, we are gaining weight. And lots of it. Recent studies show that almost two-thirds of American adults are overweight. This is a staggering statistic, one that confounds nutritionists as well as the average person who wants to maintain a healthy weight. While most Americans are scratching their heads about what and how to eat—trying to pick from the confusing array of diets that are the current rage—the reason for the epidemic of obesity in this country can be traced to one simple fact: We eat too much.

Are we a nation of gluttons? I don't think so. It's the size of our food, not the size of our appetites that's to blame. The portions, servings, helpings, slices, and amounts of what we eat have grown dramatically over the past few decades. Just look around: Everywhere you go, you are encouraged to buy huge sizes. A Double Whopper at Burger King is nearly 1,000 calories; a large order of French fries at McDonald's is 540 calories. A Double Gulp at 7-Eleven is nearly 800 calories. The jumbo bucket of popcorn at a movie theater is up to 1,640 calories. The Hungry-Man XXL frozen dinner, with a slogan that says "It's good to be full!" weighs in at 1½ pounds with 1,000 calories, a meal that packs enough heft for two. When presented with all this food, who can blame us? We can't help but eat more calories than we can burn. So we gain weight.

As the portion sizes offered to us have gotten bigger, so have we. Since I'm a nutritionist by training, I had some idea that America's collective waistline was growing, but it really hit me when I saw a dietary intake survey conducted by the National Center for Health Statistics in 1994. The shocking results? The average American adult gained eight pounds—that's eight pounds *per person*—in the 1980s. That might not sound like a lot, but compare it to earlier decades. In the 1960s and 1970s, the average weight of American adults increased only slightly, by a pound or two at most in the course of each decade. It's not just that we were heavier than ever, but we were gaining weight at a much faster rate. Why had weight gain accelerated so rapidly in such a short period of time? I knew it couldn't be genetic; the gene pool simply doesn't change that fast. What was it?

I had heard most of the reasons nutritionists were giving for the obesity epidemic—too much couch-potatoing in front of TVs and computers, changes in exercise patterns, unhealthy snacking and fast-food feasting. But I knew that these explanations couldn't possibly be the whole enchilada. I looked into the national exercise trends and found that there was virtually no change in exercise patterns during that time. So it had to be something else, something circumstantial, a change in our culture that was causing such a rapid weight gain in just three decades. I suspected that the cause was portion sizes.

I figured our national weight gain had more to do with *how much* we eat than *what* we eat. So I went to look at the research that had been done on portion sizes, to see if there was a connection between the trend toward supersized food portions and weight gain. To my surprise, there was no research. Nothing. Nobody seemed to have done any, not professors, government nutritionists, or weight-loss counselors. In fact, very few people even noticed that our food portions were growing so quickly. I couldn't find any hard-and-fast information on how big our food portions are, what portions weigh, how much they've changed over time, and how they compare to federal standards like the U.S. Department of Agriculture (USDA) Food Guide Pyramid that came out in 1992 or the Food and Drug Administration (FDA) food labels. Here I was, surrounded by nutrition experts and academics, and no one was talking about, much less studying, portion sizes.

I decided to conduct my own research. I spent a rather hot summer riding my bicycle around Manhattan, talking to deli owners, restaurateurs, and fast-food workers, asking them all sorts of questions about what they were serving and what people were eating. I became a portion detective, carrying around a food scale, a camera, and a notebook, recording the exact size and weight of typical foods that you can pick up at places around Manhattan—a vendor cart, a take-out joint, a Times Square restaurant chain, a deli—from places you grab a quick bite on the go, to a four-course sit-down dinner. What I found was appalling. I had no idea how enormous typical food servings had become. I found bagels the size of seat cushions and muffins as big as a bread loaf. I weighed different foods—street-vendor pretzels, black-and-white cookies, prepackaged muffins, and even fruits, like apples, that are closer to a cantaloupe in size and weight. I took pictures of all-you-can-eat buffets and pasta plates overflowing with pounds of noodles and tubs of sauce. I measured cups, plates, wineglasses, and margarita buckets, all gargantuan in size. I combed through *Zagat*, the popular restaurant guide, and found restaurants praised for their all-you-can-eat salad bars and buffets, free refills, two-for-ones, and troughs of pasta, all of which customers consider a selling point, with entries touting "Godzilla-sized burgers," "the biggest subs in the city," and "food piled high on the plate."

By the end of the summer, I had a big fat binder, my own "portion museum." It showed comparisons of cup, drink glass, and plate sizes; photos of obscenely large servings of pasta and meat; quotes from restaurant owners; and advertisements that lured customers with both bigger foods and bigger deals. My findings: The foods we buy today are often two to three times, even *five times*, larger than when they were first introduced into the marketplace.

portion shockers . . .

- Pizza pies were 10 inches in diameter back in the 1970s. Today Pizza Hut offers the Full House XL Pizza, a 16-inch pie. Little Caesars sells the Big! Big! Pizza, with the large measuring 16 to 18 inches with a slogan that says: "Bigger is better!" Both Pizza Hut and Little Caesars have discontinued the 10-inch pie.

- 7-Eleven stores started selling 12- and 20-ounce sodas in the early 1970s. By 1988 they were selling the 64-ounce Double Gulp, a half-gallon of soda marketed for one person.

- The famous Hershey chocolate bar weighed 0.6 ounce its first year on the market. Now the standard bar weighs 1.6 ounces, almost three times its original weight. Other sizes include the 2.6-, 4-, 7-, and 8-ounce bars. M&M/Mars increased the size of several of their most popular chocolate candy bars *four times* since 1970.

- The most popular burger places have all increased the size of their hamburgers: Burger King's original hamburger weighed 3.9 ounces, which included the bun and all. Today's Burger King burger is 4.4 ounces; the Whopper Junior is 6 ounces; and the Double Whopper is 12.6 ounces. McDonald's also started out with a pretty small patty—1.6 ounces precooked—but has upped it to the Double Quarter Pounder with 8 ounces, five times more meat. Wendy's, the chain that asked the famous question, "Where's the beef?" answered it with a triple-patty burger with 12 ounces of meat.

- Even diet food has grown in size; in the mid-1990s, Weight Watchers introduced Smart Ones, with larger portion sizes, and Lean Cuisine offered Hearty Portions, a heftier frozen dinner, with 100 more calories. The irony of diet food that advertised bigger sizes with more calories seems lost in the diet industry.

- At Starbucks the Short cup of coffee, at 8 ounces, is no longer on the menu. The smallest size is Tall, a 12-ounce cup that is nearly twice as big as what used to be considered a regular cup of coffee. Other sizes include the 16-ounce Grande and the 20-ounce Venti.

- When Chef America added 10 percent more filling to its microwave sandwich Hot Pockets while keeping the price the same, sales increased by 32 percent.

- The number of new larger-size portion sizes has increased tenfold between 1970 and 2000.

size inflation

Along with the trend toward colossal cuisine come the not-so-subtle advertising and come-ons that push us to buy bigger sizes in order to save money on food. "Bargains," "value size," and "family size" portions are everywhere. Fast-food employees are coached to suggest larger sizes and all the trimmings to customers who order small or single servings. Prepackaged supermarket foods and restaurants regularly use value as a way of pushing more food on customers.

The bigger-is-better motto that has taken over the food industry has radiated outward, affecting the size and sales of other products. Because restau-

FOOD	COMMON PORTION SIZE	
	1960	2000
BAGEL	2–3 ounces	4–6 ounces
MUFFIN	2–3 ounces	5–7 ounces
COCA-COLA, BOTTLE	6.5 fluid ounces	20 fluid ounces
CHOCOLATE BAR	1 ounce	1.5–8 ounces
POTATO CHIPS, BAG	1 ounce	2–4 ounces
MCDONALD'S HAMBURGER	1.5 ounces	1.5–8 ounces
MCDONALD'S SODA	7 fluid ounces	12–42 fluid ounces
MCDONALD'S FRENCH FRIES	2.4 ounces	2.4–7.1 ounces
PASTA ENTRÉE	1.5 cups	3 cups
BEER, CAN	12 fluid ounces	12–24 fluid ounces

portion shockers . . .

- In the course of just three years—between 1984 and 1987—the exact same chocolate chip cookie recipe on the back of the Nestlé's TOLL HOUSE Semi-Sweet Chocolate Morsels package scaled down the number of cookies it makes from 100 to 60.
- The average adult weighed nearly twenty-five pounds more yet was only about an inch taller in 2002 than in 1960 according to the National Center for Health Statistics.

rants are using larger dinner plates, you're more likely to find larger plates in stores. New models of dishwashers are designed to accommodate spaceship-size plates and bowls. Even carmakers have increased the size of standard pullout plastic cup holders to make room for larger soda bottles and take-out drink cups. If you compare the new edition of the classic cookbook *The Joy of Cooking* to the original, you'll see identical recipes for cookies and desserts. Identical in all ways except that the new recipe makes fewer servings than previous editions—16 brownies instead of 30—which means that the portions are twice as large.

The clothing industry is making clothes larger while lowering the tag size, a psychological ploy that makes more Americans the "perfect size 8." Home scales have moved the top weight readings from about 300 pounds to 400 pounds based on the demands of an increasingly obese marketplace. And the saddest, and most telling, statistic of all: caskets are now supersized. The *New York Times* reports that sales of wider, larger caskets have increased 20 percent over the past five years.

We are bombarded with huge, out-of-control portions. Maybe you noticed this already. But what are you supposed to do with this information? None of this data—the dates, percentages, and changes in portion sizes—

that I've thrown at you would matter if it didn't have any effect on our eating habits. Who cares if portions are huge, so long as they don't get in the way of eating well and maintaining a healthy weight? But they do get in the way. Big-time.

portion shockers . . .

- When Yankee Stadium was built in the 1920s, it had 82,000 seats; the remodeled version has only 49,000 seats.
- The top-selling clothing size for women jumped from size 8 to size 14 in less than 20 years.
- Those cute little Dixie cups used to be three ounces. Now the cups for cold drinks come in 21-, 24-, 32-, and 44-ounce sizes.
- The Olive Garden restaurant chain advertises the "Never-Ending Pasta Bowl," with unlimited refills of pasta, all for only $7.95.
- A glass of wine at a restaurant or a bar is most likely twice as large as it was in the 1970s.
- A queen-size bed is now 6 inches wider than it was in the 1970s.
- Restaurant diners used 26 percent more olive oil on each piece of bread as compared to butter. But the olive oil eaters ended up eating 23 percent less bread in total, so they still ate fewer total calories.

saving for later doesn't work

People eat in units, this is a fact of human nature. A cookie, a sandwich, an order of fries, a candy bar, a piece of pizza, a can of soda or beer, a soft-serve ice cream, a bag of chips. Whatever the unit is, most people will eat the entire unit, no matter how big or small. Think about it. How often do you take just a few bites of an ice cream cone, a burger, or a hot dog, and put the rest aside? Can you remember the last time you wrapped up a quarter of a slice of pizza and stashed it in the fridge for later? Or how about a soda—do you regularly cap a half-drunk bottle and keep it for another day? We may tell ourselves that we'll put the rest away for later, but who are we kidding? Remember the ad for Alka Seltzer with the memorable tag line, "I can't believe I ate the whole thing." Everyone can relate to that feeling of not being able to stop until the entire package is gone.

A lot of people would never order a second helping of something—two frozen yogurts, another popcorn bucket, one more order of fries—but have no problem buying a medium of any of these foods (which is usually twice as large as a small) and finishing the whole thing. Presented with two smalls or one medium, they almost always think that they're eating less with the medium portion because one serving *must* be less than ordering a second helping. My client Jane always orders a medium frozen yogurt but would never dream of buying two smalls for herself, even though the medium is exactly the same size as two smalls combined.

Elaine, a fifty-five-year-old professor, told me that she wanted to cut back on eating an entire Balance bar. She wanted a few bites to tide her over between meals, but she knew that she didn't need to eat the whole thing. Only problem was: She couldn't stop eating it. She always finished it, against all of her instincts and desires. So I suggested she switch to Pria bars, which are about half the size of Balance bars. She switched and now eats half the size without feeling like she's missing out on anything. Again, it's just easier to eat an entire unit—in this case, a Pria Power Bar—than to eat half and save the rest for later. In fact, Pria has started advertising it as the "perfect-size" snack. This time the advertising is on target, though I'd prefer you have a piece of fruit, fresh vegetables, or low-fat yogurt as a snack.

bigger portions mean you eat more

An important study conducted by Pennsylvania State University researchers shows that we eat more when larger food portions are plunked down on the table. Exactly how much more do we eat? It turns out to be 30 to 50 percent! That means when we sit down and are given a huge amount of food, such as an overflowing pasta bowl that's too large

1976   7-Eleven sells 16-oz Gulp
   •   Hershey's Milk Chocolate Bar weighs 1.4 oz
1977   Soft-drink industry begins using 2 liter bottles
1978   7-Eleven adds 32-oz Big Gulp
   •   Between the Bread introduces oversized muffins
1979   Pizza Hut adds 13-inch pie
   •   Hershey's replaces 8-oz and 16-oz cans of Hershey's chocolate syrup with 24-oz bottle

1980 - 1984
1980   Hershey's Big Block chocolate bars
   •   M&M/Mars increases size of Snickers, M&Ms, Three Musketeers, and others
1981   M&M/Mars markets King-size M&Ms
   •   Hershey's Milk Chocolate Bar now weighs 1.5 oz
   •   Hot and Crusty Bakeries sell oversize muffins
1982   M&M/Mars increases size of candy bars again
   •   Burger King adds Bacon Double Cheeseburger
   •   46-oz movie popcorn introduced (32-oz discontinued)
   •   85-oz movie popcorn introduced
1983   Taco Bell introduces Nachos BellGrande
   •   7-Eleven 44-oz Super Big Gulp
   •   Pizza Hut's Personal Pan Pizza (larger than single slices)
1984   Some movie theater chocolate candy bars have increased by 25%—Nestlé Crunch (3.5 oz) and Reese's (3 oz)
   •   Chocolate candy bars increase in size—AGAIN!
   •   Pizza Hut's Big Topper Pizza (a third larger than Personal Pan Pizza)
   •   Well-Bred Loaf distributes oversized muffins.

- *Veryfine apple juice introduced in 11.5-oz cans, up from 10-oz bottles*
- *Wendy's "Where's the Beef?" campaign*
- *Chicago Metallic, a distributor of commercial baking pans, introduces oversized muffin pans*
- *Jumbo-size stadium pretzel is introduced*

1985–89

1985 *Movie-theater candies increase in size—Juji Fruit is 7 oz instead of 3 oz*
- *32-oz movie soft drink introduced*
- *Howard Johnson's sandwiches increase to 3.5 oz*
- *Howard Johnson's burger increases to 4 oz*
- *New larger sizes of Cracker Jack introduced*
- *McDonald's "Large Fries for Small Fries" promotion*
- *McDonald's increases Large fries to 4.5 oz (former Large now called Medium)*
- *Wendy's adds Big Bacon Classic*

1986 *130-oz movie popcorn introduced*
- *Big Apple Bagels, a national bagel chain opens with 5-oz bagels*
- *Dunkin' Donuts introduces 4-oz bagels*
- *Regular Hershey's bar reaches its highest weight of 1.7 oz*

1987 *44-oz movie soft drink introduced*
- *Hershey's introduces King-size Reese's Peanut Butter Cup*
- *Manhattan Bagel Company, a national bagel chain opens*
- *Toll House chocolate chip cookie recipe yields 60 cookies (instead of 100)*

1988 *Taco Bell announces free drink refills*

to eat in one sitting, we routinely eat 30 to 50 percent more than we would if we were handed a smaller plate. What's even more surprising is that, even though we eat more, we don't feel more full. We feel the same as if we had a smaller serving. Furthermore, we usually don't make any adjustment in the next meal, eating less because we happened to overeat earlier in the day, or yesterday. It's almost as if that huge meal never existed! It's interesting to note that when the researchers conducted similar studies with toddlers, they found that three-year-old children stopped eating when they were full. But as soon as children reach age five, they will continue to eat, even after being full, just like an adult. Clearly, there is a pattern of overeating when presented with more food that begins in childhood. Parents, take note.

portion distortion

The supersizing of American food has caused many of us to suffer from "portion distortion." We've all become so accustomed to gargantuan servings that the terms "small," "medium," and "large" make no sense anymore. We no longer have any way to judge how much we eat. I asked students in my nutrition classes at New York University (NYU) to bring in what they considered a "medium"-size apple, baked potato, bagel, muffin, and cookie. They were surprised to find that every single item they brought in was larger than a "medium" as it's defined by federal standards. In most cases it was twice as large.

portion shockers . . .

- Women ate 31 percent more (159 more calories) and men ate 56 percent more (355 calories) when served a 12-inch sub sandwich instead of a 6-inch sandwich.
- When asked to take out spaghetti from different size boxes to make dinner for two, women took 302 spaghetti strands when given a 2-pound box but only 234 strands when given a 1-pound box. One ½-cup serving of pasta is 32 spaghetti strands.
- When frying chicken, women poured 4.3 ounces of cooking oil from a 32-ounce bottle but only 3.5 ounces from a 16-ounce bottle.
- When people were asked how many M&Ms they would eat when watching a movie by themselves, they poured about twice as much from a jumbo bag (63 from a small package and 103 from a package double the size), a difference of about 250 calories.
- Moviegoers who said that the popcorn tasted stale still ate 61 percent more than when given a larger container than a smaller one. Even when it doesn't taste great, people still eat more out of a large container.

American portion distortion is clear when you compare U.S. portions to their European counterparts. Pasta is usually an appetizer in

- McDonald's adds Super-Size soft drink
- McDonald's adds Super-Size fries
- Wendy's sales increase due to serving larger burgers
- McDonald's sells Medium Fries
- 7-Eleven 64-oz Double Gulp
- Lance introduces larger 4.5-oz and 7-oz sizes of potato chips, corn chips, and tortilla chips
- 10- and 16-oz Tropicana Twister beverages
- Bagel Oasis makes bigger bagels along with everyone else in late 1980s
- Bagels now weigh 4 to 6 oz, up from 1.5 to 2 oz when first introduced in US by Jewish bakers from Poland
- Movie-size 4-oz Kit Kat (up from 2 oz) introduced

1989   Wendy's Biggie Fries introduced
- Wendy's Biggie drinks introduced
- M&M/Mars King-size Milky Way

1990–1994

1991   Hormel introduces 10.5 oz micro-cup products (up from 7.5 oz) for several products (including lasagna and noodles with chicken)
- Beech-Nut introduces 7.5-oz microwaveable meals for toddlers, competing with Gerber's 6 oz
- American Home Products' Chef Boyardee Main Meals— 6 different entrees
- Consumer promotion at movie theaters: "large soda and large popcorn, get free candy bar"
- Hershey's Big Block bars are renamed King-size
- 170-oz movie popcorn introduced
- ConAgra adds extra portion offerings to Healthy Choice line

- *Muffin tops introduced—even the tops alone are big*

1992 *Swanson's Hungry-Man frozen dinners weigh 15 oz*

- *Healthy Choice adds Extra Portion dinners*
- *Lender's sells Big 'N Crusty bagels*
- *Oscar Mayer Big and Juicy hotdogs added*
- *24-oz Arizona iced tea introduced*
- *Heineken 21.6-oz bottle introduced*
- *Thomas sandwich-size English muffin, 63% larger than regular size*
- *Pillsbury Grands! Biscuits introduced—40% larger than other items*
- *Pillsbury Sweet Rolls increase by 30%*
- *Little Caesars Pizza by the Foot*
- *Nestlé introduces King and Giant Size bars; offers three sizes of Nestlé Crunch bars (1.55-oz Regular, 2.75-oz King, and 5-oz Giant); markets the Butterfinger Beast (5-oz bar with nearly 700 calories)*
- *M&M/Mars King-size Twix*
- *Restaurant dinner plates grow to 12.5 inches*

1993 *McDonald's Mega Mac*

- *Howard Johnson increases weight of burgers and sandwich meats*
- *Domino's Dominator*
- *Frito-Lay introduces Super-size potato chips and Doritos (20 oz)*
- *Pizza Hut Big Foot Pizza*
- *20-oz Coca-Cola adds plastic bottle*
- *Heineken introduces 24-oz bottle (replaces the 21.6 oz)*

1994 *"Get Your Burger's Worth" campaign"; Burger King increases hamburger patty and other items by 50%*

restaurants in Italy, where several swirls of a fork will finish off an entire plate of fettuccine. Cappuccino can be found only in one small size. This is the reason that my client Jackie routinely loses twenty pounds every time she takes her annual summer trip to Europe. I hear this over and over again from American tourists in Italy: "I ate all the time—pasta, cheese, bread, even pizzas—and still lost weight." The reason: They are eating less because the portions are much smaller.

down with calorie counting

Here's the bottom line: No matter what you eat, no matter how healthy it is, no matter what the label says—dietetic, low-fat, no-carb—the bigger the size, the more calories it has. And if you eat more calories than you burn, you gain weight. It doesn't matter if you eat low-fat, fruit-sweetened bran muffins until the cows come home; if you're eating ten of them a day, you're going to gain weight.

Expanding portions sizes is the primary reason that we are facing an obesity epidemic. Calories add up quickly when the portion sizes are so large. Nutrition authorities recommend that we eat approximately 2,000 to 2,600 calories a day to stay the same weight, while older, sedentary women, and young children should have a bit less and active men and teenage boys a bit more. To put this in perspective, a breakfast bagel and a slice of pizza add up to nearly half of the calories recommended for an entire day. Once you add the cream cheese, a soda, and dinner at a Chinese restaurant, your calorie count for the day can easily top 3,000.

But who can look at food and know how many calories are in it? Nobody, not even the experts. I was asked by the Center for Science in the Public Interest (CSPI), a consumer advocacy group in Washington, D.C., to study how accurately dietitians are able to judge the calorie content of different restaurant meals. We showed 200 dietitians five plates of food that are actually served in restaurants—lasagna, a Caesar salad with chicken, a tuna salad sandwich, a porterhouse steak platter, and a hamburger with onion rings. We asked the dietitians to tally up the damage, and guess what? Although they were all seasoned professionals, they had no idea how many calories were in these foods. Some underestimated the calories by as much as half.

When Marian Burros, a renowned food and nutrition writer for the *New York Times*, heard about the experiment, she decided to put four experts—Dr. Marion Nestle, my NYU thesis advisor (and now Paulette Goddard Professor of Nutrition); Dr. Isobel Contento, chair of Columbia University Teacher's College program in nutrition; Gaynelle Clay-Williams, then a doctoral candidate at Columbia and obesity researcher at St. Luke's–Roosevelt Hospital; and me—in the hot seat. We were given eight heaping plates of fatty food and were quizzed on the calorie and fat content. It was a disaster. We were all over the place with every single dish, either under or over on calories or fat. Not one of us was remotely on

- Wendy's Great Biggie Fries
- McDonald's MBX (Big Extra)
- Burger King's Big King
- Hardee's promotes Monster Burger with two quarter-pound patties, 3 slices of cheese, and 8 strips of bacon
- Jack in the Box launches the Ultimate Cheeseburger with two quarter-pound patties, 3 slices of cheese, and 4 strips of bacon
- The newest edition of The Joy of Cooking features recipes for monster cookies and jumbo muffins; recipes that used to yield six servings now yield four
- United Airline tests bigger portions
- Annual soft-drink consumption jumps to 56 gallons, up from 21 gallons in 1970
- The number of fast food restaurants per capita doubled since 1972
- The King-size Goldenberg's Peanut Chews chocolate bar increases from 2.7 oz to 3.3 oz
- Jamba Juice, a chain store of juice bars, offers 24-oz blended fruit drink containing over 500 calories.

1998   M&M/Mars offers a 3.7 oz Snickers Bar (The Big One), 76% bigger than the regular size
- Hershey's advertises its Milk Chocolate Bar with the tag line: "14% free—get an 8-oz bar at the 7-oz price"
- T.G.I.Friday's menu offers margaritas in "huge 18-oz goblets," "two thick 8-oz" pork ribs, and a "hefty helping" of mashed potatoes
- Applebee's advertises a riblet platter that is "over a pound" and a "hearty portion" of chicken fingers

target. If the nutrition experts can't figure out the calories in a restaurant meal, who can?

This is why calorie counting is useless. It works only in a completely controlled environment with carefully weighed and calibrated food. We are not lab rats. We do not eat and live in a sealed-off bubble, like the space shuttle, where calories are measured by laboratory analysis. If you eat at a restaurant for only one meal of the day, you have completely lost count of your calorie intake. This was the case with my client Barb. She came to me with stacks of index cards that were filled with the calorie count of each and every meal she had, whether at home, on the run, or at a restaurant. Little did she know that the counts weren't accurate. She was only fooling herself into thinking she was sticking to a strict calorie regimen.

Not only was Barb incorrect in her assumptions about calories, she was buried in index cards, calculations, and calorie charts. This dedication to calories may work for a while, but for most people, it's not a way to live. It's cumbersome, time-consuming, and a bit neurotic. Working with me, Barb started estimating portions and eating a nutritionally balanced diet. And she finally did lose weight—nearly seventy pounds—not because she was counting calories, but because she became more *aware* of how much she was eating.

With all of our obsessive calorie counting, you would think that we would have a deep understanding of how the *size* of foods relates to the calorie content. Not so. I work with Larry, a very educated, successful fifty-year-old man who wants to lose that last ten pounds. I met him in his ele-

reality check— more food = more calories!

FOOD	MANUFACTURER/ EATING ESTABLISHMENT	CALORIES/ REGULAR SIZE	CALORIES/ LARGE OR JUMBO SIZE
SOFT DRINK, BOTTLE	Coca-Cola	100 cal/8 fluid ounces	250 cal/20 fluid ounces
FRENCH FRIES	McDonald's	210 cal/Small (2.4 ounces)	540 cal/Large (6.2 ounces)
HAMBURGER SANDWICH	Burger King	320 cal/ Hamburger (4.4 ounces)	920 cal/ Double Whopper (12.6 ounces)
M&MS	Mars Inc.	240 cal/regular size (1.7 ounces)	770 cal/movie megasize (5.3 ounces)
COFFEE FRAPPUCCINO	Starbucks	180 cal/Tall (12 fluid ounces)	300 cal/Venti 20 fluid ounces)
ICE CREAM, VANILLA	Häagen-Dazs	270 cal/1 scoop (½ cup)	810 cal/3 scoops (1½ cups)
FROZEN YOGURT	TCBY	110 cal/kiddie cup (3 ounces)	350 cal/Large cup (11 ounces)
POPCORN (POPPED IN OIL)	Movie theater	400 cal/small 7 cups	1160 cal/large 20 cups
CINNAMON BUN	Cinnabon Inc.	300 cal/ 3-ounce Minibun	670 cal/ 8-ounce Cinnabon

Sources: Manufacturers, Center for Science in the Public Interest, U.S. Department of Agriculture.

- Sizzler restaurants offer a 24-oz steak
- California Pizza Kitchen increases 9-inch pizzas to 10 inches; adds 3 oz to pasta dishes
- Value-sizing program at Lamb Weston
- Boston Chicken adds more sides
- Weight Watchers Smart Ones meals now come in larger portions
- Tasty Baking Company introduces a five-item Snak Bar line of baked goods: larger 2-oz cookies compared to usual 1.3- to 1.5-oz
- Lender's Bagel Shop bagels— bigger and better than ever
- Restaurants now offer "towers of flavor," piling greater and greater height on the plates
- Miller introduces 20-oz and 1-liter single-serve plastic bottles for Miller Lite, Miller Genuine Draft, and Icehouse
- Burger King tests new slower-cooking broilers to accommodate thicker chunks of beef
- Burger King offers Small (2.6 oz), Medium (4.1 oz), and King (6.1 oz) French fries

1999 Loews movie theaters offer free refills
- The Lone Star Café features the 72-oz Steak Challenge, "which separates the men from the boys," free to anyone who can finish it, along with its trimmings, in less than one hour
- Burger King test-markets Great American Burger
- Heineken introduces 16-oz beer can
- Mrs. Fields' introduces Stokabunga, a 5-oz "energy boosting" cookie

gant office on Madison Avenue, where I go over his eating habits, looking for ways that he can painlessly cut back on his portion sizes. We were talking about a subject that I try to avoid—calories—when he asked a question that stunned me: "You know I like frozen yogurt. Does a medium have more calories than a small?" Now, let's take a moment to think about Larry's question. He is asking, essentially, whether a bigger size has more calories than a smaller size. The answer is a resounding yes. *Always.* Unless you are talking about plain water, black coffee, or diet soda, more of anything that you consume has more calories. When I say that a Double Gulp has nearly 800 calories, people act shocked. How can that be? they wonder. Simple: It is eight times bigger than an 8-ounce soda, which has 100 calories. I cannot stress this enough: *Larger portions contain more calories.* The chart on page 19 shows how more food means more calories. It's just math.

And finally, one single slice of carrot cake at the Cheesecake Factory contains a whopping 1,560 calories. That's because it's a 14-ounce slice!

Do you need to count calories? The answer is no, you don't need to count calories. You are going to learn how to estimate portions. You are going to understand the food groups and the healthiest options from each group. This is the most important information you will ever need to eat nutritiously and to achieve and maintain a healthy weight. Wanda, a nurse practitioner in her forties, was shocked when she heard me say that she never had to count calories again. She told me how easy it was going to be, and she was right; she started losing weight and was thrilled with the simplicity of it. With a little practice, you'll stop carrying around that calorie chart, or counting up the calories of your dinner, or looking at a cookie as a number. Soon you'll just see another portion.

portion shockers . . .

- Carl's Jr. introduced the "double $6 burger" in 2004 which contains an entire pound of beef and 1,400 calories.

- The average amount of beer consumed by men over forty has increased from 23 to 32 ounces, a switch that results in about 100 more calories.

- Upsizing a Minibon to a classic Cinnabon costs only 24% more but contains 123% more calories, according to the National Alliance for Nutrition and Activity.

- Switching from a 6-inch to 12-inch tuna sub at Subway costs only 47 percent more but has 100 percent more calories.

- The French croissant doubles in size when baked in America.

down with diets

Diets don't work. I know you have heard this before—in women's magazines, in diet books, from weight-loss counselors—but you may not under-

* Solo Cups now sells 46-oz cups, quite a difference from the 1950s when the 7-oz was the only size available
* Automakers introduce larger adjustable cup holders to accommodate giant drinks
* McDonald's increases the weight of Super-Size fries by nearly one ounce; the former Super-Size is downgraded to a Large, and the Large becomes a Medium
* Burger King begins test-marketing the half-pound Great American hamburger
* McDonald's introduces the 42-oz Super-Size drink; the 32-oz Super-Size is downgraded to Large

2000–2004

2000 Pizza Hut introduces The Big New Yorker, a 16-inch pizza
* 7-Eleven introduces the Big Brew, a 24-oz cup of coffee (Need a jolt?)
* Hershey Foods introduces the Big Kat, a full 27% bigger than the regular Kit Kat
* Kraft markets bigger Lunchables Mega Pack for kids
* Dainty demitasse cups replaced with oversized mugs
* Sweetheart Cup Company sells 24-oz hot-beverage cups
* Restaurant reviews frequently mention portion size; Zagat's NYC restaurant guide features entries for Godzilla-sized burgers, Fred Flintstone portions, and bathtub-size hero sandwiches

2001 Average home is 2,324 sq feet, up from 1720 sq ft in 1981
* Even though Burger King Large fries was phased out in 1998 in favor of the King, the company decides to make the King bigger by nearly an ounce (6.9 oz), and add the Large size, weighing 5.7 oz

- Burger King introduces a 42-oz King drink
- Swanson enlarges its Hungry-Man line of frozen dinners with the XXL, containing 1½ pounds of food, up from the early 1990s where the meals weighed slightly under a pound (not that they were ever small!)
- Banquet, a company boasting "America's #1 Frozen Brand" of turkey dinners introduces "Double the Meat" entrees in its new Hearty One line of meals
- Nike adjusts sizing of women's clothing; what used to be Medium is now Small
- Average refrigerator increases to 28.6 cubic feet from 19.6 in 1980
- Shaquille O'Neal pitches Burger King's meaty-cheesy-bacony-X-treme Whopper (but he exercises a lot!)
- Jack in the Box beefs up its burgers by 66% without raising prices; also begins using larger patty for Jack's Kids Meals for an extra 10 cents
- Wendy's markets the Classic Triple with Everything, including 3 slices of cheese, which weighs 14.5 oz and has 1,030 calories
- Crate and Barrel sells more charger plates as dinner plates
- Top-selling clothing size for women is now size 14, compared to size 8 in 1985

2003
- Pizza Hut makes 12-inch Medium, 14-inch Large, and 16-inch Big New Yorker
- Burger King drops Small fries
- Hardee's restaurants debuts Thickburgers, a line of hefty sandwiches weighing ⅓ pound, ½ pound, or ⅔ pound

stand why and that there is a rational and healthy alternative. All diets are based on the assumption that you "go on" them, meaning you change your eating habits for a short period of time, after which you can return to "normal." And too many diets are based on crazy claims; it seems that all common sense goes out the window when it comes to dieting.

I came to the weight-loss world with a broad interest in health, not from a single, somewhat narrow "one-size-fits-all" diet plan. First as a manager of a weight-loss center and later as a nutrition counselor for weight-loss programs and an obesity researcher.

I've never been a fan of strict food plans, regimented eating programs, and diet trends. I have never, ever had one client count calories. What I offer is a plan, not a diet. Most programs simply tell you to cut forbidden foods completely. I know you may be willing to do that for a while, but I doubt you can do it forever. Can you, or better yet, *should* you stop eating all carbohydrates forever if you don't want to? Absolutely not. Fad diets such as high-protein and high-fat regimens help you lose weight in the short run because they exclude entire food groups or nutrient categories from your diet, which translates into less calories per day. These diets may help you lose weight temporarily, but they rarely address the real problem, and that problem is the larger *sizes* of our food portions, along with our total lack of understanding of what constitutes a reasonable "portion."

On this program, I'll teach you how to smart-size your portions. You will learn about food groups, standard serving sizes, how many servings you should eat per day, and how many servings from each food group your meals actually contain. There are no restricted foods. You can eat from any food group during the day, as long as you balance your portions and make informed decisions. On my program, there's no going "on" or "off," no yo-yoing back and forth, from abstinence to "everything goes," no switching from grapefruit to low-cal Jell-O to all-you-can-eat steak and eggs. My program offers a healthy way of life without deprivation. It incorporates all your favorite foods and the way you like to eat. There is no sense of guilt, or cheating, or throwing it all out the window. You can start at any time, any day, to eat well and live healthfully. You do not have to walk around with a food scale and a measuring cup, nor do you have to add up points. Instead, you will retrain your eye and learn a completely new way of thinking about what you eat.

Nothing gives me more pleasure than watching someone hit their ideal weight while learning and having fun. Over the years I have helped many clients—both adults and children, male and female—develop healthy eating habits and lose weight while continuing to dine at their favorite restaurants and eat foods they love. After working together for several months, Bea, a thirty-eight-year-old doctor who wants to lose a total of eighty pounds, said, "This just can't be possible. This is too easy. This doesn't even feel like a diet." The reason is that it's *not* a diet. It's an eating plan. And it sure has worked for Bea.

* Burger King now has five sizes of burgers, toppings and all: the 4.4-oz Hamburger, the 6-oz Whopper Jr., the 6.1-oz Double Hamburger, the 9.9-oz Whopper, and the 12.6-oz Double Whopper (with nearly 1000 calories); Burger King opened with 3.9-oz burger

* Denny's introduces bigger entrees: a massive breakfast for $4.99, The Meatlover with 2 eggs, 2 sausages, 2 bacon strips, ham, hash browns, and 3 pancakes

* IHOP sales increase with Stuffed French Toast

* IHOP introduces giant-size Super Stackers sandwiches

* Jumbo-size Kellogg's Raisin Bran box is 25.5 oz, up from original 15-oz box in 1942

* McDonald's Super-Size Value Meal, a Quarter Pounder with cheese, fries, and a Coke contains 1550 calories

* Kraft introduces Easy Mac Big Pacs with 50% more macaroni and cheese

* McDonald's offers four sizes of fries: Small (2.4 oz), Medium (5.3 oz), Large (6.3 oz), and Super-Size (7.1 oz)

* Nestlé promotes a 1.75-oz Crunch bar with the label slogan: "10% more than the 1.55-oz bar"

* Hershey Foods introduces the Reese's Peanut Butter Big Cup, one large 1.5-oz cup

* Hershey Foods offers ToGo, convenient single-serve, 2.75-oz bags of chocolates such as Mini Kisses, Kit Kat, and Reese's Bites

* Hershey Foods markets 12-oz bags of individual snack-sized chocolates, weighing 0.6 oz each, which just happens to be the exact same size as the original chocolate bar introduced in 1908

Bea, like so many of us, loves a number of "pleasure" foods that she doesn't want to, or can't, give up: peanut butter, nuts, rice, and corn flakes. She has lost a total of forty-two pounds and is more than halfway toward her target weight. On the Portion Teller program, Bea can have her peanut butter and eat it, too! The trick for Bea (and for you, too) is that she eats sensible portions of the foods she loves, instead of cutting them out entirely and feeling deprived.

The other important point about Bea's story is that she has set reasonable weight-loss goals. Rather than focus on the total amount of weight she has to lose—an impossible-sounding eighty pounds!—she focuses on smaller losses, one step at a time. She knows that any weight loss is better than the all-or-nothing approach. Research also shows that losing even small amounts of weight leads to improved health. In fact, a colleague of mine in the nutrition world needed to lower her cholesterol. She lost ten pounds in three months and her cholesterol went down eighty points. Small changes like this can make a world of difference. The proof is in the pudding. Small, everyday, and even simple changes lead to big results. The first step toward a lifelong change in your eating habits is portion-size awareness, the foundation of the Portion Teller program.

- *Hershey's Milk Chocolate Bar now available in 1.6-oz, 2.6-oz, 4-oz, 7-oz, and 8-oz sizes (Quite a difference from the original 0.6-oz bar! The smallest bar is more than 3 times the original size and the largest bar is more than 13 times the original size!)*
- *M&M's at movie theaters weigh 5.3 oz*
- *7-Eleven replaces the 16-oz size with the 20-oz Gulp; other soda sizes available are 32 oz, 44 oz, and 64 oz*
- *McDonald's drink sizes: 12-oz Child, 16-oz Small, 21-oz Medium, 32-oz Large, and 42-oz Super-Size*
- *Hardee's and Carl's Junior introduce big, low-carb bunless burgers, often containing ½ pound of meat wrapped in lettuce (You'd be better off with a small burger and a bun! Sorry!!)*
- *Wal-Mart carries "extended sizes," meaning XXL and the like*
- *Kohl's carries pants with expandable waists; Croft & Barrow Flexon Model contains 4 full inches of extra belly room*
- *Average bra size is 36C, up from 34B in 1991*
- *Average woman's shoe size now 8½, a full size larger than 15 years ago and four sizes bigger than the 4½ women wore at the turn of the century*
- *Grocery stores are expanding. Kroger's grocery store now contains 25,000 square feet. Why? To accommodate MORE food!*
- *Average bus seat is 18 inches wide, up an inch from 1997*
- *Pottery Barn sells 12-inch dinner plates*

making sense
of standards

It's a Monday morning. You pick up your regular pint of juice on your way to work. Then you start to wonder: It's one carton. How does this translate into how much fruit you should be eating in one day? When you get to work, you look up the government's Dietary Guidelines for Americans on the Web. It tells you that for an average diet you should have 2 cups (4 servings) of fruit per day. You think . . . 2 cups. That's a pint, isn't it? Did I just eat all my fruit? Then you turn to the Nutrition Facts panel on the carton itself. It says that the carton contains 2 servings of juice. But that's not 4 servings, it's only 2. So can I have an apple this afternoon? Should I? What does it all mean?

You're really trying to do the right thing, but at this point, you're so frustrated that you give up. Why try to quantify what you're eating when it's so hard to figure out what's "right"?

This scenario, which I guarantee is happening all over the country, all the time, shows how confusing serving size information is, especially as it relates to nutrition education, food labels, and calorie charts. Why is this information, which was intended to make it easier to choose a healthy diet, so difficult to decipher? And, more to the point, does it resemble in any way our dietary reality, or how much we really eat? There are three federal standards for servings

- New dishwashers can accommodate oversized plates
- Scales now accommodate a hefty weigh-in of 400 pounds, up from 300, until recently the industry standard
- Coffins are larger; traditional casket was 22.5 inches wide, Goliath Casket's new triple-wide is 44 inches wide
- Pets are fatter. So are bears. They are eating our leftovers...
- Americans spend $110 billion on fast food—up from 6 billion 30 years ago
- Queen-size beds contain an extra 6 inches
- Mattress sizes have increased; standard full-size is 53 by 75 inches, California King is 72 by 84 inches

2004 Stage Deli launches the "Hugh Jackman," a triple-decker sandwich five inches high containing a pound of meat (corned beef, turkey, pastrami, and roast beef), cheese, and 3 bread slices

- Steelcase makes a desk chair that holds 500 pounds
- Morristown introduces a rocking chair/recliner big enough to hold a small family: it measures 4 feet across, holds 600 pounds, and includes a motorized lift
- Cookietree Bakeries markets a "quarter pound mega bite" oatmeal cookie, which is more like an oat-meal than a cookie
- McDonald's announces plans to phase out its Super-Size French fries and soft drinks. The largest order of fries will be the Large weighing in at 6.3 oz (as opposed to 7.1 oz), the same weight as the Super-Size fries 5 years ago. The largest drink size will be the 32 oz Large, a quart of soda.

- *Carl's Jr unveils "double $6 burger" Containing an entire pound of beef (three times the meat recommended for an average adult over the entire day)*
- *Hardee's introduces the Monster Thickburger—two 1/3-pound slabs of Angus beef, four strips of bacon, three slices of cheese, and mayonnaise on a buttered sesame seed bun—packing 1,420 calories and 107 grams of fat; with fries and a soft drink, this single meal would involve more calories and fat than most people should get in an entire day*
- *The Centers for Disease Control and prevention announces that due to the increasing weight of Americans, U.S. airplanes consumed an extra 350 million gallons of jet fuel in 2000, costing the airline industry $275 million a year*

sizes—the USDA Food Guide, the FDA food labels, and the USDA Nutrient Database for Standard Reference, the primary source of food composition data, including calorie and nutrient content of commonly consumed foods. These three guides can be confusing or useful. Here's what you need to know.

the usda food guide

You've seen it, maybe on the back of a box of crackers. It looks so simple—but what are you supposed to do with it? The USDA Food Guide Pyramid that has been the nation's nutrition standard since 1992 says that we're supposed to eat at least 6 grain servings per day. What does that mean? How much is that? It sounds like we can eat bread all day long. If you look at the actual size of the Pyramid servings according to the USDA definitions, you understand 6 servings. One serving of pasta isn't a deep-dish trough. It's ½ cup cooked—that's 32 strands of spaghetti—or the size of a handful (yours, not Muhammad Ali's).

The government released new guidelines in 2005 that attempt to clarify the confusion over serving sizes. The sixth edition of the Dietary Guidelines for Americans emphasizes cups and ounces over servings. For example, the guidelines recommend that the average person eat "6 ounce-equivalents" of grains per day. What is an equivalent? According to the guidelines, 1 ounce is "equivalent" to a slice of bread, ½ cup of cooked pasta, or 1 cup of cereal flakes. Confused yet? Who knows how much food weighs (in ounces or grams) or how that relates to volume (in cups or teaspoons)?

In the Dietary Guidelines, some of the portion definitions are surprising. For example, a "small" muffin is defined as 1 ounce, which is more like a quarter of the average muffin top alone, and considerably smaller

portion shockers . . .

- Sizzler offers the "granddaddy of them all," a 24-ounce porterhouse steak. Steak lovers beware—this steak contains more than three days' worth of meat according to USDA recommendations.
- A typical muffin weighs in at over 6 ounces and comprises more than an entire day's worth of grains recommended for many Americans by the Dietary Guidelines.
- Some deli sandwiches contain 1 pound of meat, about three days' worth of meat recommended by the USDA.
- In a survey conducted by the American Dietetic Association, more than 50 percent of people overestimated a standard serving size of pasta.

than most "mini" muffins available in the marketplace. The Food Guide can be useful, however, if you're motivated enough to look for and read the materials that the USDA publishes. And the good news is that the 2005 Dietary Guidelines stresses more fresh fruit, vegetables and whole grains.

food labels

You would think that food labels would list the exact same serving sizes as the Pyramid. It sure would make things easier. No such luck. The FDA used different criteria to determine standard serving sizes for food labels than the USDA did for its Food Guide, so they differ in many cases, even though many people assume that they're the same. According to the USDA guidelines, a serving of pasta is ½ cup cooked. But according to the FDA food labels, a serving of pasta is 2 ounces dry, which translates into 1 cup cooked—twice as much. There's no getting around it: Glaring discrepancies exist between the FDA food labels and the USDA Food Guide.

Almost everyone who is watching what they eat takes a look at food labels for one reason or another. That's all fine and good, but the single most important piece of information on any food label is the serving size. It's the basis for all of the other data: calories, nutrients such as carbohydrates, fat, sodium, and so on. So start with the serving size, then look at the number of servings per container or package, and multiply or divide according to how much you plan on eating. If you eat the entire package, multiply all of the calories and nutrients by the number of servings. Sounds simple, but you would be surprised how often people are thrown by this information. If the package is big, like a party-size bag of potato chips, you usually don't forget to multiply. But if the package is small, it still may contain two, three, or even four servings. Tons of packages are marketed as single serving sizes, but when you look closely at the label, it turns out that it's two or three servings. Pretty sneaky, huh? Who hasn't been on a diet and made a nice meal with a bed of lettuce, some tomato wedges, a little lemon juice, and a 6-ounce can of tuna on top? Perfect meal for one? Yes, it actually is—despite the label on the tuna can, which says it contains 2.5 servings. This silly labeling has gotten so out of hand that the FDA has announced plans to require food companies to list calories and nutrition information for the entire package. Several food manufacturers, including Coca-Cola, have already announced plans to make such revisions immediately.

Another important point about food labels: If you are buying a product that's made by a small, regional company, even one that sells "health food," the labels are often notoriously inaccurate. To prove this, I conducted a study of prepackaged baked goods, like brownies, muffins, and cookies. I weighed them and then compared the actual weight with the label weight. The information on the label consistently underestimated the true weight of the food, often by as much as 25 percent. You can't trust the label—another reason you need to be aware of portion size.

calorie charts

Calorie charts are derived from the USDA food composition table, known as the Nutrient Database for Standard Reference. Surprise, surprise, the serving sizes that are the basis for the calorie charts are often quite small and don't reflect what we're offered in restaurants and fast-food joints. Take a slice of pizza. The USDA table lists it as 2.3 ounces (140 calories), whereas an average slice is about 7–8 ounces. People don't understand that they may have to multiply the calories found in the charts by at least 3 or 4 to get an accurate read. It's hard to blame the USDA. Portions are increasing so quickly that it can't possibly update the charts fast enough. Just remember: Calorie charts are accurate only for the weight information provided. If you have no idea how much your food weighs, the calorie counts will be incorrect. In fact, a huge discrepancy exists between how much we say we eat and how much we really eat. Consider this: The United States food supply produces 3,900 calories per person per day, but the average person reports eating far less. (According to the most recent survey, women report eating 1,877 calories and men report eating 2,618 calories.) Where's all that extra food going? While some of it is going into the garbage, a lot is going into the stomachs of people who can't tell how much they're eating.

a serving versus a portion

With all the confusing information out there, how can a person who is concerned about eating healthfully sort through it all? Before we go any further, it's important that you understand the difference between a *serving* and a *portion*. I call a *serving* a standard unit of measure, whereas I use *portion* to talk about how much food you actually eat. Your portion may contain several servings. When I tell people that the serving size of a salmon steak is 3 ounces, or about the size of a deck of cards, they say, "You don't think I'm actually going to eat a piece of fish that's as small as a deck of cards?" to which I respond, "No, I don't. But I want you to know *how many* decks of cards you have on your plate and how many you're eating." What you put on your plate is a portion, not a serving. Distinguishing between a portion and a serving is the start of gaining portion-size awareness.

Now that you have a sense of how important it is to pay attention to how much you eat, it's time to get to the nitty-gritty. *The Portion Teller* teaches you how to eat healthfully and happily for the rest of your life. You'll learn nutrition basics and how to use visuals to evaluate your portions. You'll figure out your own Portion Personality, keep a food diary for a short time. and learn how to improve your food plan with Smartsize substitutions. Ultimately, you'll come away with easy-to-follow ways to smartsize your life.

• get smart! •

- Start paying attention to serving sizes on the labels of foods you eat regularly.
- Forget about saving for later. Buy one portion at a time.
- Don't fall for sales ploys that say "Bigger is better."

the portion teller visuals

*My doctor told me to stop having
intimate dinners for four, unless there
are three other people.*

• ORSON WELLES

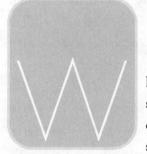

hat happens when people are told their daily meals should include 6 oz. of grains, 5.5 oz. of meat, 2.5 cups vegetables, 6 teaspoons of oil, and so on? Ever seen anyone pull out a food scale at your favorite restaurant? I doubt it. Most people just assume that 6 ounces means six servings and that they can have six bread items every day. What Americans usually don't take into account is the *size* of the grain servings. Take a look at a typical person's daily grain consumption:

- bagel for breakfast (5 grain servings)
- sandwich for lunch (2 grain servings)
- pasta for dinner in a restaurant (6 grain servings)
- one single-serving oatmeal cookie as a snack (4 grain servings)

This typical pattern adds up to 17 servings from the grain group (or, by the government's definition, 17 ounce-equivalents). In reality, if you eat 1 bowl of pasta in a restaurant, 1 muffin, or 1 bagel, you've had all your grains for the day. There's no question that we're eating too many carbs. But that doesn't mean we need to cut all carbs from our diets, including fruits, vegetables, and healthy starches such as sweet potatoes and whole-grain breads. When it comes to dieting, we seem to have a psychological need to simplify everything to one common denominator—cut out all carbs, eat only grapefruit, have as many nuts as you want all day long—the list goes on and on, changing with the latest fad. We want to believe in a magic pill or some miraculous way to trick our bodies into losing weight by eating strange combinations of foods. But how can you follow this "magical formula" for the rest of your life, restricting yourself to one type of food or mixing together a bizarre combination of foods? What happens when you go out to eat or travel? What happens at a cocktail party or when you get hungry while you're shopping? This approach just doesn't work over the long haul—life intervenes, and the diet goes out the window.

If you cut out or lean too heavily on any one food group, it's more difficult to obtain key nutrients and have a well-rounded diet. Even if you don't know what these nutrients do for you, I'm sure you know that it's a good idea to get your daily dose of them. And it's much better to get them from real foods than to get them from a vitamin.

Another drawback to getting rid of an entire food group is that you often overeat from other groups. Joan, a client in her mid-forties, figured that she could live without dairy and got rid of it, preferring to get her calories elsewhere. But during the day, especially in the late afternoon and late evening, she got hungry, and ended up nibbling on extra bread and turkey, more than making up for the calories she saved from the dairy group.

We need to eat less food from all food groups, instead of cutting out carbs. And we need to eat better. But how do we do that? With the Portion Teller three-pronged program: *nutrition awareness, portion-size awareness,* and *self-awareness.* This chapter is all about nutrition and portion-size awareness. Once you've got this information under your belt, you will know how to eat the *right* foods, in the *right* amounts, at the *right* times in order to manage your weight and feel satisfied. There's a lot to absorb here, but remember: This isn't a fad. This is what you need to understand to eat healthfully for the rest of your life!

the portion teller
weight-loss pyramid

Let's get down to basics—nutrition basics, that is. Meet the Portion Teller Pyramid. The Portion Teller Pyramid is the basis for a balanced, healthy food plan that allows you lose weight and keep it off. It gives you almost all you need to know about nutrition without the index cards, flash cards, scales, and calorie charts. A clear understanding of the different food groups is the basis of a balanced diet. The Portion Teller Pyramid introduces you to six food groups—(1) Vegetables; (2) Fruits; (3) Grains and Starchy Vegetables; (4) Fish, Poultry, Meat, and Meat Alternatives; (5) Dairy; (6) Fats; and Treats and Sweets, the tiptop section of foods that you should eat sparingly since they aren't part of a balanced diet.

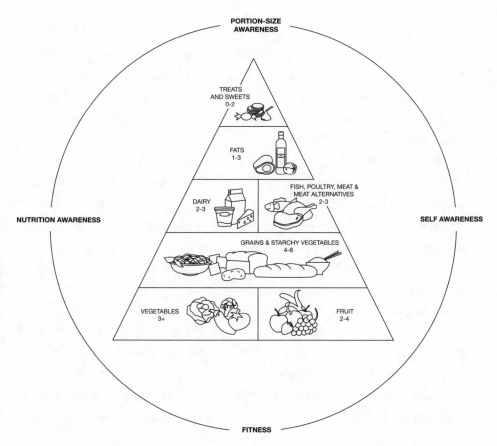

Take a close look: The Portion Teller Pyramid breaks food down into food groups and says how many servings from each group that you should eat each day for a balanced diet. Built into this pyramid are these main concepts: Eat lots of fruit and vegetables. Don't overdo it with grains, where portions tend to be huge. Low-fat dairy is nutritious. Meat servings are smaller than you think. And there is a place for fats and sweets—I'll show you how to incorporate them. See how each food group has a number of daily servings? What is a serving? We know it's not what's on your plate—that's a portion! We know calories are too hard to count. And we're certainly not carrying around a food scale. So let's figure out what the servings on the Portion Teller Pyramid really are.

sizing up servings

The buffet table, the cocktail party spread, the all-you-can-eat salad bar: they are every dieter's nightmare. You walk up to them with an empty plate, and before you know it, you've piled on all sorts of food—who knows how much—and then you're back for seconds and thirds. The problem with this kind of eating is that no one can tell how much they're putting on their plates and into their mouths.

Consider peanut butter. How often can you say that you opened a jar of peanut butter and started scooping and eating, scooping and eating, until you've eaten half the jar? The serving size on the label is 2 tablespoons, which is something like ⅟₁₆ of a normal jar. How could anyone possibly figure out what ⅟₁₆ of a jar is without dumping the jar out and dividing it up? This is hardly the most convenient way to eat peanut butter. So how can you tell how much food you're about to put in your mouth? You need to size up your servings, and here's how. It's a piece of cake.

I'm going to show you a variety of foods, the kind you probably eat all the time, and compare their serving sizes to some simple, everyday objects: a CD case, a deck of cards, a walnut, a golf ball, a baseball, a tennis ball, a shot glass, a matchbook, a cap on a water bottle, a standard postage stamp, a computer mouse, a CD, and an Altoids tin. Let's size it up: 2 level tablespoons of peanut butter looks like a whole walnut in its shell. If you know this, you'll be hard-pressed next time you take three or four huge scoops to say that you have no idea how much you ate. You'll know that you're having, say, 3 walnuts worth, or 6 tablespoons, which is probably too much to have in one sitting. You'll be able to tell you've gone overboard long before the bottom of the jar starts peeking out under the peanut butter. In the case of cheese, 1 ounce equals 4 dice. This is especially helpful if you're eating cheese that is cut into cubes, the way it often is at cocktail parties. You need to connect what's on your plate with easily recognizable units of measure. So instead of talking about ½ cup of rice, because most people can't figure out how much that is, you can think in terms of ½ baseball. You need to size up your servings.

After a little practice you'll be able to associate standard amounts, like ½ cup, with an everyday object and its size. You can estimate how much is on your plate whenever you eat, whether you are at a party or a restaurant or in your own kitchen. At home, it's easier. When you're serving yourself, you have a real-life frame of reference to help you decide how much to put on your plate. You can check the serving sizes on the box, follow the servings in a recipe, or even use a measuring cup on occasion, but you can't do that when you're eating out. By sizing up servings, you will *know* how much you're eating in every situation. Getting used to these visuals forces you to pay attention to your portions. My clients tell me all the time that they never look at food in the same way again—I've ruined their ability to eat with abandon. They know too much.

Visuals are easy to relate to what you eat. When I ask someone to describe the size of a sandwich he had for lunch, inevitably he'll rattle off every single detail about a sandwich he had days ago: whole-grain bread; no mayonnaise, but a little pesto sauce on piece of the bread; a few sprouts; sun-dried tomatoes; Monterey Jack cheese; and turkey. But when I ask how much turkey or cheese, or how big the sandwich was, he is always completely stumped. He'll give me a confused look and say, "It was an average-size sandwich." But there is no such thing as an "average" anything when it comes to food. It's all relative. But when I ask people to compare the amount of turkey they had to some recognizable item, they light up and say, "Yes, about as much as a deck of cards in each half sandwich." Eureka! Few people, other than professional chefs and very experienced home cooks, truly understand food weights, but *everyone* can relate to visuals.

visuals

Do you have any idea what 1 ounce looks like? These pictures of common foods next to everyday objects will help you estimate *how much* of something you're eating. This has nothing to do with what you should eat or what a standard serving size is. These visuals simply help you judge *measurements*. Once you're able to judge a measurement, you can tell exactly how much is on your plate. For instance, you may not be able to estimate the size of 3, 6, or 9 ounces of meat, but you can probably answer the question: How many decks of cards are on my plate: 1, 2, or 3? Photocopy these visuals and carry them with you until you get used to them. In the next chapter, you'll learn how many servings these visuals represent.

Visualizing Food

Meat or poultry; fish such as tuna or salmon steak	*3 ounces = deck of cards*	
Fleshy white fish, such as flounder, sole, etc.	*3 ounces = checkbook*	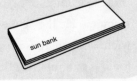

Meat or poultry	*1 ounce = matchbook*	
Peanut butter	*2 tablespoons = walnut in the shell*	
Salad dressing	*2 tablespoons = shot glass*	
Olive oil or salad dressing	*1 teaspoon = standard cap on a 16-ounce water bottle*	
Butter or margarine	*1 teaspoon = standard postal stamp*	
Cold cereal; berries; popcorn	*1 cup = baseball*	
Rice or pasta, cooked	*½ cup = ½ baseball*	

Ice cream	½ cup = ½ baseball
Tomato sauce	½ cup = ½ baseball
Pretzels (1 ounce)	¾ cup = tennis ball
Bread (1 ounce)	1 slice = CD case
Pancake/waffle	4-inch diameter = diameter of a CD
Hard cheese	1 ounce = 4 dice
Cheese slice, sandwich meat	1 ounce = diameter of a CD

Baked potato or sweet potato	*1 potato = computer mouse*
Mixed nuts; dried fruits; granola, almonds, or peanuts	*¼ cup = golf ball*
Juice, orange or grapefruit (6 fluid ounces)	*¾ cup = 6-ounce yogurt container*
Apple, peach	*1 piece of fruit = baseball*

THE HANDY METHOD

Sometimes the best visual to use is your own hand. The Handy Method helps you guesstimate your portions by comparing your foods to different parts of your hand. Sure, everyone's hand is a different size, but if your hand is smaller than average, you probably are smaller than average and need less food. To go back to the cheese example, you may not have a set of dice with you at all times, but you always have your hand. To figure out how much cheese you've just picked up (or wolfed down, as the case may be), all you have to do is hold it up to a finger—your index finger will do. If the cheese is about the same size as your finger, you know you have around 1 ounce. If you've eaten or put more "fingers" of cheese on your plate than you have on your hands, you're getting awfully close to an entire pound of cheese.

Take the cocktail-party dish of nuts—the kind of food you could care-lessly nibble on all night and end up overeating without even knowing it. Not with the Handy Method. Since you probably don't have a golf ball on you, just grab a bunch of nuts and spread them over your palm. One single layer of nuts equals about ¼ cup—no cheating and doubling allowed! All you have to do is put the nuts in your hand before eating to estimate your portion. Don't fall into the trap of just picking at nuts straight from the dish. Before you know it, the entire dish is empty.

And one more food trap—the movie theater, with its bottomless buckets of popcorn. Just grabbing piece after piece adds up quickly, especially if you're watching a movie and absentmindedly digging into the bucket. If you want an idea of how much you're eating, scoop out 1 rounded handful. That's about ½ cup. Or cup both your hands together and scoop out a mound of popcorn. That's a cup.

The Handy Method

Meat, fish, or poultry	3 ounces = palm of your hand	
Mixed nuts	¼ cup = 1 layer on your palm	
Veggies, berries	1 cup = tight fist	

Popcorn/cereal	1 cup = 2 cupped hands or 2 handfuls	
Cooked pasta	½ cup = rounded handful	
Meat, cheese	2 ounces = 2 fingers (length of 2 fingers) 1 ounce = 1 finger	
Butter or oil	½ teaspoon = fingertip	

Rules of Thumb

Peanut butter, butter	*1 teaspoon/thumb tip*
Peanut butter	*1 tablespoon/3 thumb tips*
Meat, cheese	*1 ounce/thumb*

portion-size awareness

Honestly, did you ever have any idea what an ounce really looked like? Now you do. Whether you use the Handy Method or the visual comparisons, sizing up servings makes you mindful of exactly how much you're eating at any time. No more eating with ignorance. You will have developed your own "internal" portion-size awareness that you can take with you wherever you go, in any situation. Once you have this knowledge, you're in control of exactly how much you eat. That's a major step. So now let's put it to use.

food groups and
serving sizes

To lengthen thy life, lessen thy meals.
• BENJAMIN FRANKLIN

n this chapter, I'm going to tell you more about each food group and show you how much you should be eating. It contains a complete chart of the serving sizes of most foods in all the food groups. This chart is also in Appendix D. You can turn to it for easy reference as you teach yourself about the foods you like to eat. So don't memorize. Just try to absorb the different food groups, paying special attention to the serving sizes and the number of servings in each food group and keeping an eye out for your favorite foods.

portions and servings

A Reminder: Don't forget the difference between a portion and a serving. To return to the example that I've been using throughout the book, a bagel is 1 portion. But just because a bagel is 1 portion, or 1 unit, doesn't mean that it's 1 serving. Let's end the bagel myth once and for all! By now you may remember that a typical bagel is actually 5 grain servings. Portion-size awareness, the number-one goal of learning how to smartsize, is the ability to estimate how many servings (or standard units) are in your portion (what you actually eat).

Some notes: Whenever I'm dealing with a prepackaged or single-serve item like a bagel or muffin, I use the realistic or typical size that you find in stores. But that still doesn't mean you should eat the whole thing. For foods that are not preset sizes, such as rice, meat, fruit, fruit salad, and so on, I settle on simple, easy, usable units of measure. A few examples: A serving of cooked rice is ½ cup (½ baseball or 1 handful). A serving of fresh fruit salad or mixed berries is 1 cup (1 baseball or 1 tight fist). A serving of cooked chicken is 3 ounces (1 deck of cards or your palm). A serving of yogurt is 1 cup (an 8-ounce yogurt container). The units are always standard and easy to multiply or divide; I don't make you get out the calculator for 1⅛ cups of a food or suggest something atypical, like 2 teaspoons.

HOW BIG IS A CONTAINER OF YOGURT?

Single-serve yogurt used to always come in an 8-ounce container. Then some manufacturers decided to cut costs by making 6-ounce containers. Now some yogurts are 8 ounces and some are only 6. Should you worry about the extra 2 ounces? No. Eight ounces of low-fat yogurt is full of calcium and protein. It's a healthy serving of dairy. Just opt for low-fat or nonfat varieties and don't worry about which size you're buying. Worry about the bigger chocolate bars and soda bottles, not the yogurt.

The serving sizes and visuals that follow are a guide for you to use to develop portion-size awareness. Once you've got the basics under your belt and start to incorporate it into your daily eating, I promise that you won't have to go back to it again and again. It will become part of your new, healthy approach to portion control.

• reality check—nutrients •

What is a "nutrient"? Nutrients are components of foods that help nourish the body. There are six categories: proteins, carbohydrates, fats, vitamins, minerals, and water. Protein, carbs, and fats are energy-yielding nutrients, meaning that they provide calories that give you energy to move about your day. Vitamins, minerals, and water don't give you energy or provide calories.

We all know some foods are better for you than others, but which ones, and why? Skim milk is better than oozey, gooey Brie, but they're in the same food group. Whole-wheat toast has got to be better for you than a gigantic muffin, but they're also in the same food group. The key is nutrient density. Technically speaking, nutrient density is a measure of the nutrients provided per calorie of food. Stated more plainly, it means getting the most nutrient bang for the buck, a good nutrient value for the least amount of calories. So even though cheddar cheese, ice cream, and crème fraiche are all dairy products, they don't all have the same caloric or nutritional value as yogurt, skim milk, or low-fat cottage cheese. Under each food group, I list the Smart Bets, the most nutrient-dense choices. With nutrient-dense foods, you don't have to worry if you eat a little too much. If you splurge on blueberries or broccoli, your jeans will still fit you tomorrow. Below are several examples of nutrient-dense varieties of commonly consumed foods.

FOOD	NUTRIENT-DENSE VARIETY
bagel	whole-wheat bread
French fries	baked potato
hamburger	turkey breast
ice cream	low-fat yogurt
pineapple juice or dried pineapples	fresh pineapple

fruits and nonstarchy vegetables

Fruits and vegetables are the base of the Portion Teller Pyramid. That's easy to remember because fruits and vegetables are the foundation of a healthy diet. I suggest 2 to 4 fruit servings and 3 or more vegetable servings a day. Fruits and veggies are the optimal choice for dieters, for anyone who wants to eat healthfully, and for growing kids. They are low in calories and chock full of vitamins, minerals, fiber, phytonutrients, and antioxidants, such as vitamin C in oranges and lycopene in tomatoes.

Do you have to cut fruits and vegetables from your diet because they contain carbohydrates? Feel free to post this statement on your fridge and take a good, hard look at it every time you open the door for a snack: *No one ever got fat from eating too many carrots!*

Besides the health benefits, veggies are great for dieters for another reason: They make you feel full. They're loaded with water, which makes you feel as if you've eaten more than you actually have. The other reason you feel fuller, faster, on a diet loaded with veggies is that they contain fiber.

• reality check—fiber •

Get this: Fiber is the only food component that the body doesn't digest. That means it contains no calories. Even so, eating foods rich in fiber makes you feel full. When you feel full, you eat less. Fiber can be found in fruits, vegetables, whole-grain breads and cereals, and starchy vegetables (like potatoes, but not potato chips or French fries). It would be silly to cut out fiber when you're trying to lose weight. Besides filling you up without making you fat, fiber is beneficial to your overall health: It aids in digestion, helps keep you "regular," contributes to the overall well-being of your digestive tract, and may reduce the risk of certain diseases, such as diverticular disease, heart disease, and certain cancers. Although meat can be tough and hard to chew, it contains *no* fiber. Nor do these foods contain much fiber: white-flour products (bagels, white bread, white-bread crackers, and most muffins), candy, soda, and all sweets.

NONSTARCHY VEGETABLES:
3+ servings daily

Good news. Nonstarchy vegetables are totally free. Starving? Go for it. Fill up. Have as much as you want. It's important to choose a variety of veggies. Just make your plate pretty. Eating a rainbow of colored vegetables will bring you different phytonutrients that have health benefits. (The deep-orange color of carrots indicates that they provide the antioxidant beta carotene.) **Note: Starchy vegetables such as corn and potatoes are categorized in the grain group.**

1 cup raw = 1 baseball
½ cup cooked = ½ baseball

Alfalfa sprouts

Artichokes

Asparagus

Bamboo shoots

Bean sprouts

Beets

Broccoli

Brussels sprouts

Cabbage

Carrots

Cauliflower

Celery

Cucumber

Eggplant

Fennel

Green beans

Greens (collards, kale, mustard, turnip)

Kohlrabi

Leeks

Mushrooms

Okra

Onions

Pea pods

Peppers (red, yellow, green)

Radishes

Salad greens (arugula, endive, escarole, assorted lettuce, romaine)

Scallions

Snow peas

Spaghetti squash

Spinach

Sugar snap peas

Summer squash (yellow or zucchini)

Tomatoes

Water chestnuts

Watercress

Salsa, ½ cup	½ *baseball*
Tomato sauce, tomato puree, ½ cup	½ *baseball*
Tomato juice, 1 cup (8 fl. oz)	*1 baseball*
V8 juice, 1 cup (8 fl. oz)	*1 baseball*
Vegetable soup, 1 cup (8 fl. oz)	*1 baseball*

Smart Bets: *All veggies, especially a colorful assortment. Nutrition superstars include asparagus, broccoli, carrots, red peppers, and spinach.*

Limit: *There's no need to avoid any vegetables. They are ALL good for you.*

A Note on Preparation: *On the Portion Teller plan, nonstarchy vegetables are free, but fat isn't. If you cook your vegetables, try steaming or microwaving. If you do grill or sauté your vegetables, make sure you pay attention to how many servings of fat you use and tally them with your daily count.*

FRUIT:
2 to 4 servings daily

Fruit is loaded with stuff that's good for you. As with vegetables, a variety of colors will bring you a variety of nutrients. But fruit does have sugar in it, so sticking to 2 to 4 servings is best. If you're a real fruit lover, it's okay to cheat a little here—the fiber in the fruit should fill you up before you go too far. That's why you should limit fruit juice. You can guzzle a whole container without feeling full.

Apple, 1	*1 baseball*
Applesauce, unsweetened, 1 cup	*1 baseball*
Apricots, fresh, 4 whole	
Banana, 1	
Berries (blackberries, blueberries, raspberries, strawberries), 1 cup	*1 baseball*

Canned fruit, unsweetened, 1 cup	*1 baseball*
Cantaloupe, 1 cup	*1 baseball*
Cherries, fresh, 1 cup	*1 baseball*
Clementines, 2	
Dried fruit, ¼ cup (e.g., 9 dried apricots, 4–5 prunes, small box of raisins, 2 dried figs)	*1 golf ball*
Figs, fresh, 2	
Fruit juice: orange, grapefruit, cranberry, 6 fl oz	*6-oz yogurt container*
Fruit salad (assortment of mixed fruits), 1 cup	*1 baseball*
Grapefruit, ½	
Grapes, 1 cup	*1 baseball*
Honeydew, 1 cup	*1 baseball*
Kiwi fruit, 2	
Mango, ½, or 1 cup	*1 baseball*
Nectarine, 1	*1 baseball*
Orange, 1	*1 baseball*
Papaya, ½, or 1 cup	*1 baseball*
Peach, 1	*1 baseball*
Pear, 1	*1 light bulb*
Persimmon, ½, or 1 cup	*1 baseball*
Pineapple, fresh, 1 cup	*1 baseball*
Plums, 2	
Tangerines, 2	
Watermelon, 1 cup	*1 baseball*

Smart Bets: *All fresh fruits. Nutrition superstars include blueberries, kiwi fruit, citrus, and melons.*

Limit: *fruit juices, dried fruits, canned fruits in syrup*

• reality check—sugar •

Like carbs, sugar has gotten a bad rap recently. But also like carbs, that reputation is not entirely fair or correct. Not all sugars are bad for you. But do stick with the ones that occur naturally in food. These include sugar found in fruits, vegetables, and dairy. The unhealthy sugars are added or are concentrated sugars, such as those in candy, soft drinks, and sweets. Limit: sucrose (table sugar), corn syrup, fructose, glucose, maltose, high-fructose corn syrup, maple syrup, honey, and molasses. Simple, isn't it?

grains and starchy vegetables: 4 to 8 servings daily

Grains of all kind—rice, bulgur, couscous, oatmeal, pasta, bread, popcorn, crackers, cereal, and so on—form the next level of the Portion Teller Pyramid, with 4 to 8 servings each day. Be careful with grains. White flour products, such as bagels and muffins, have increased in size over the past few decades, sometimes as much as *400 percent*. Don't be deceived by what you're served or buy when it comes to grains—more so than any other food group, grains are the biggest part of the supersize movement.

Opt for healthy grains. I provide a long list of healthy choices from the grain group: items made from whole wheat, rye, or oats. The less-nutritious grains are easy to spot; they are white-bread products, such as white bread, muffins, bagels, pasta, and so on.

• reality check—carbohydrates •

My client Sharon, a twenty-eight-year-old advertising executive, fell victim to the carb myth. She was absolutely convinced that certain vegetables are "fattening" and the cause of her weight problem, so she avoided them like the plague. But at the end of the day, she found herself feeling hungry and unsatisfied after eating a diet based entirely on protein, so she turned to the starches—chips, crackers, and bread products—to fill her up. I explained to her if she only had some water- and fiber-rich fruits, like a peach or some juicy melon slices, or a nice plate of asparagus or cauliflower with a splash of olive oil, she would end the day feeling full, with no need to binge on the bread. When Sharon changed her habits, she was able to lose weight while filling up on lots of healthy fruits and vegetables.

Murray, a thirty-nine-year-old banker, wanted to lose about twenty pounds. When we first met, he had a whole list of questions about carbs. He was convinced that every single food containing starch was out. He even asked if fruits and vegetables are starches. I explained to him that some vegetables—potatoes, corn, and beans—are "starchy," and are similar to bread in calories and carbohydrate content, but all fruits and most vegetables aren't starches. And the ones that are, such as sweet potatoes with their skin, corn, and beans, are quite good for you. Murray was thrilled to hear that a baked sweet potato with his fish or chicken at dinner or a bowl of oatmeal for breakfast is not off limits; in fact, it's a great diet choice.

This is why I consider it my nutritional duty to rehabilitate the carbohydrate and its bad reputation. Let's set the carb record straight. All fruits, vegetables, beans, grains/starchy vegetables, and dairy (yes, dairy) foods contain carbohydrates. These carbohydrates eventually break down or convert into, among other things, sugar, technically known as glucose, which has 4 calories per gram. A carb is a carb is a carb when it comes to calories. But not when it comes to nutritional value; a cookie and a carrot may both have carbs, but they obviously don't offer the same health and diet benefits. In other words, *all carbs are not nutritionally equal.* Some are much more healthy for you than others. Don't stop eating broccoli, carrots, and oranges. It's just crazy. When people eliminate fruits and vegetables from their diets, they miss out on vital nutrients: fiber, vitamins such as folate and vitamin C, and minerals such as potassium.

The healthy ratio of proteins, carbs, and fats in your diet is as follows: 10 to 35 percent protein, 45 to 65 percent carbs, and 20 to 35 percent fats. The Portion Teller Pyramid falls into this range. Try to incorporate nutritious carbohydrates into your diet and to spot which carbs are nutritious—the good guys—and which ones are less nutritious.

NUTRITIOUS CARB CHOICES

- Fruits
- Vegetables
- Healthy starches:
    Whole grains, including whole-wheat, rye, and oat-bran breads
        and cereals, brown rice, barley, bulgur, kasha
    Starchy vegetables: sweet potatoes, corn, baked potatoes,
        winter squash, beans
- Low-fat diary: nonfat and low-fat milk, and yogurt

NON-NUTRITIOUS CARB CHOICES

- White-flour products, including white bread, bagels, crackers, cookies, cakes, muffins
- Foods/drinks with added sugar: candy, sodas, sugar-sweetened drinks, sugary cereals

Note that on this program, starchy vegetables like potatoes, corn, peas, winter squash, and beans, aren't in the vegetable group. They're here, in the grain/starchy vegetable group. And no, you can't eat unlimited quantities of them. Technically, a potato is a veggie; it grows in the ground. But it has a similar calorie and macronutrient—carbohydrates, protein, and fat—content to a slice of bread. With this in mind, you can substitute half a baked potato for a slice of bread. French fries, which the government classifies as a vegetable, accounts for one-fourth of American's vegetable consumption. No wonder we're overweight. I put French fries at the tip of the pyramid, in the Treats and Sweets category.

Beans and legumes are a terrific food choice. They're classified as starchy vegetables and contain lots of fiber, vitamins, and minerals. Yet they also contain protein, making them a preferred meat alternative for vegetarians. Are beans fattening? Beans fall into the same category as bananas, watermelon, and carrots: No one ever got fat from eating too many of them. And you won't find yourself overdosing because they're loaded with fiber. When you smartsize, you can count beans in either the starchy vegetable food group or the meat alternative group. You decide. Just choose one.

STARCHY VEGETABLES

Cassava (yucca), ½ cup cooked	½ *baseball*
Corn, 1 ear	
Corn, ½ cup cooked	½ *baseball*
Green peas, ½ cup cooked	½ *baseball*
Legumes (beans, peas, lentils),* ½ cup cooked	½ *baseball*
Black-eyed peas, black beans, chick peas (garbanzo beans), kidney beans, lentils, lima beans, pinto beans, split peas, white beans	
Parsnip, ½ cup cooked	½ *baseball*
Plantain, ½ cup cooked	½ *baseball*

*NOTE: Legumes can also be counted as a meat alternative. Do not count in both groups.

Potato, baked with skin, ½, about 3–4 oz, or ½ cup	**½ computer mouse**
Potato, boiled, ½ cup	**½ baseball**
Pumpkin, ½ cup cooked	**½ baseball**
Rutabaga, ½ cup cooked	**½ baseball**
Sweet potato, yam, baked, ½, about 3–4 oz, or ½ cup	**½ computer mouse**
Winter squash (butternut, acorn, pumpkin), 1 cup cooked	**1 baseball**

WHOLE GRAINS OR HEALTHY GRAINS

Amaranth, ½ cup cooked	**½ baseball**
Barley, ½ cup cooked	**½ baseball**
Bread slice, whole-grain (whole-wheat, rye, oat), 1 oz	**CD case**
Bulgur (tabouli), ½ cup cooked	**½ baseball**

Cereal:

ready-to-eat (cold) unsweetened cereal, whole-grain, approximately 1 oz

Puffed wheat or puffed brown rice, 2 cups	**2 baseballs**
Flakes (bran, corn, oat), 1 cup	**1 baseball**
Oat rings (Cheerios), 1 cup	**1 baseball**
Brown rice cereal, 1 cup	**1 baseball**
Shredded Wheat (1 biscuit)	
Spoon-sized Shredded Wheat, ½ cup	**½ baseball**
Low-fat granola, nuggets, muesli, ¼ cup	**1 golf ball**

Cooked cereal:

whole-grain, ⅔ cup cooked (⅓ cup uncooked or 1 packet)	**1 tennis ball**
Buckwheat groats, ⅔ cup cooked	**1 tennis ball**
Cracked wheat, ⅔ cup cooked	**1 tennis ball**
Oat bran, ⅔ cup cooked	**1 tennis ball**
Oatmeal, ⅔ cup cooked	**1 tennis ball**
Wheatena, ⅔ cup cooked	**1 tennis ball**

Cereal or granola bar, whole-grain, 1, 1 oz

Couscous, whole-wheat, ½ cup cooked　　　　　　　　　　*½ baseball*

Crackers, whole-grain varieties, 1 oz　　　　　　　　　　*CD case*

　　　　2–3 large (size of whole-grain crispbread such as
　　　　　　Ryvita, Kavli, Finn Crisp)

　　　　2–3 breadsticks, whole-wheat, approx 4½ in

　　　　5–6 small (size of whole-grain Wheat Thins)

Kasha (buckwheat groats), ½ cup cooked　　　　　　　　*½ baseball*

Matzo board, whole-wheat, 1

Millet, ½ cup cooked　　　　　　　　　　　　　　　　　*½ baseball*

Pancake, whole-grain varieties, 1 (1 oz or
　　approx 4 in across)　　　　　　　　　　　　　　　　*diameter of CD*

Pasta, whole-wheat, ½ cup cooked　　　　　　　　　　　*½ baseball*

Pita, whole wheat, 1 (1 oz or approx
　　4 in across)　　　　　　　　　　　　　　　　　　　*diameter of CD*

　　　　Pita, large, 2 oz = 2 servings

Popcorn, air-popped (microwave, no fat added), 3 cups　　*3 baseballs*

Pretzels, whole-wheat or oat-bran,
　　1 ounce (¾ cup, small bag)　　　　　　　　　　　　*1 tennis ball*

Quinoa, ½ cup cooked　　　　　　　　　　　　　　　　*½ baseball*

Rice, brown or wild, ½ cup cooked　　　　　　　　　　　*½ baseball*

Rice cakes, 2 regular size (4 in) or 10 mini　　　　　　*diameter of 2 CDs*

Soba noodles, ½ cup cooked　　　　　　　　　　　　　*½ baseball*

Tortilla, whole-wheat, 1 oz (7-in)

　　　　Large tortilla, 2 oz = 2 servings

Waffle, whole-grain varieties, 1 (1 oz or approx
　　4 in square)　　　　　　　　　　　　　　　　　　　*diameter of CD*

Wheat germ, 3 tbsp　　　　　　　　　　　　　　　　　*1½ walnuts*

• reality check—
single servings •

Bagels, muffins, street (soft) pretzels, and knishes, are very large and contain several servings.

What is 1 serving of these foods? 1 ounce. That equals:

- ⅙ average-size muffin (bran, corn), ½ mini muffin, ½ muffin top, 1 bite-size muffin (1 muffin = at least 6 bread servings)
- ⅙ street-vendor hot pretzel
- ⅕ bagel, ½ scooped-out bagel *(Note:* Half a bagel is a single serving only if it's half of a mini-bagel—the ones that are the size of a yo-yo!)
- ¼ knish (potato, kasha)
- ½ English muffin, ½ hamburger bun, ½ bialy, ½ kaiser roll, ½ dinner roll

White-Flour Products

Sliced white bread, pita, tortilla, waffles, pancakes, cereals (the same serving sizes for whole grains apply here)

Crackers: 1 oz   **CD case**
   2–3 large crackers (size of graham crackers)
   2–3 breadsticks
   5–6 small crackers (size of saltines)
   8 animal crackers
   24 oyster crackers
Pasta (spaghetti, macaroni, lasagna noodles), ½ cup cooked   **½ baseball**
Pretzels, 1 oz (¾ cup)   **1 tennis ball**
   1 Bavarian/Baldie
   2 pretzel rods
   9 three-ring, 20 mini-twists
   48 sticks
Rice, white, ½ cup cooked   **½ baseball**
Taco shells, corn, 2 (6-inch)

Smart Bets: *whole-grain breads and cereals (whole wheat, rye, oat), cooked cereal, such as oatmeal and Wheatena; brown rice, kasha, bulgur, barley; all starchy vegetables, such as sweet potatoes, corn, winter squash; legumes such as lentils, chick peas, and kidney beans*

Limit: *white-flour products, such as white bread, pasta, bagels, crackers, muffins, pretzels, white rice; cereals with added sugar; and, of course, beware of giant-size bread products*

Healthy Hints: *Pay special attention to single-serve items that are available in huge sizes: muffins, bagels, scones, street pretzels, and knishes. Even if you're buying "brown" bread, you can't be sure it's made from the whole-wheat flour. Always read the label for the words "whole wheat" before buying "health" bread products.*

• reality check—white, wheat, or whole wheat: what's the difference? •

Here's a quick lesson on the difference between white and whole-wheat products. All bread comes from the same source: a kernel of wheat. White bread has been refined, stripped of the healthy parts, and bleached white. What's left is the starch, devoid of fiber and many beneficial vitamins and minerals. Whole-grain or whole-wheat flour is not refined; the entire grain is left intact—fiber, nutrients, and all. That's why whole-grain breads are much healthier. But beware: Just because bread is brown doesn't mean it's made of whole-wheat flour or that it is healthier. Brown bread often is colored with molasses and other added ingredients. In other words, it's dyed brown to make it look like it's good for you. Check the label to make sure that the ingredient list begins with *whole* wheat or *whole* grain, not just wheat flour. Food labels list ingredients in the order of their predominance in the product; that is, the earlier an ingredient is listed, the more of it there is. If wheat flour and sugar are listed up front, that means they are the predominant ingredients, so stay away, even if the bread has that "healthy" dark color.

fish, poultry, meat, and meat alternatives: 2 to 3 servings daily (approx 6 to 8 ounces)

The meat group is a terrific source of protein. The good news about protein is that a little of it goes a long way toward making you feel full. Try to incorporate a small amount of protein into each meal. What is a small amount? One serving. The palm of your hand. There are lots of lean sources of protein, found mostly in the meat and dairy groups: chicken breast, turkey, game, seafood, fish, beans, eggs, low-fat yogurt, cheese, and milk. Eating a serving of lean protein at each meal makes you feel satisfied with relatively few calories. Ever try to be good by having a green salad for lunch, only to find that, by late afternoon, you're hungry for something a little more "solid"? Afternoon cravings disappear when you add a small amount of some lean protein to your lunch. And you don't need to eat an entire cow to feel satisfied. My client Jane feels so much more satisfied after adding 2 to 3 slices of turkey or a small can of tuna to her chopped salad—and so will you!

The Portion Teller Pyramid recommends 2 to 3 meat servings a day and stresses fish, poultry, and healthy meat alternatives such as legumes (beans, peas, lentils), soy (including tofu, tempeh, and soy burgers), and eggs. I suggest you choose an assortment of healthy fish at least twice a week, especially salmon, tuna, and sardines, which contain omega-3 fatty acids, a healthy, beneficial fat that is not found in red meat. Be sure to vary your assortment of fish. And watch not only how much you eat, but also how you prepare it: Grill, broil, or bake your fish instead of frying it. Limit red meat to once or twice a week. And watch your portion size.

Nuts are a source of protein. But since nuts and nut butters, such as peanut butter, have so much more fat than meat for a similar protein content, I've taken the peanut butter out of the meat group and placed it with nuts in the fat category.

And finally, try to include one meat alternative a day, if possible. These alternatives add a lot of volume to your diet for relatively few calories. Chop up an egg or throw about ½ cup of chick peas onto your salad, and you have the protein equivalent of only 1 ounce of turkey or chicken. And it beats diet boredom.

3 ounces cooked/1 deck of cards
NOTE: 4 ounces raw yields 3 ounces cooked

Beef

Chicken

Cornish hen

Fish (bass, cod, grouper, haddock, halibut, ocean perch, red snap-
per, salmon, sardines, sole, swordfish, tuna)

Game (buffalo, venison)

Lamb

Liver

Pork

Seafood (scallops, shrimp, lobster, oysters)

Turkey

Veal

MEAT ALTERNATIVES

Eggs, 2–3	
Egg substitute, ½ cup	
Egg whites, 4–6	
Hummus, ½ cup	*½ baseball*
Legumes (beans, peas, lentils),* 1 cup cooked	*1 baseball*
Bean (split pea, white bean) or lentil soup, 1 cup	*1 baseball*
Soy/veggie burger, 1 (3 oz)	*1 deck of cards*
Textured vegetable protein, 3 oz	*1 deck of cards*
Tofu or tempeh, 1 cup	*1 baseball*

*NOTE: Protein in 1 oz meat/fish/poultry = 1 egg, 2 egg whites, ½ cup cooked legumes)

Smart Bets: *poultry (without skin), fish, and meat alternatives. Include leaner cuts of beef (USDA Select or Choice grades, trimmed, such as round, sirloin, and flank steak; tenderloin; roast; T-bone)*

Limit: *processed sandwich meats such as salami, bologna, sausage; hot dogs; bacon and spareribs*

Healthy Hints: *Try to eat a little bit of protein with each meal (with the emphasis on "little").*

Don't pile all your meat for the entire day into one meal—spread it out during the day.

Limit red meat to once or twice a week. And watch your portions!

Don't eat more than 2 servings of fish, poultry, or meat (6 ounces cooked) at one sitting.

Try to have fish at least twice a week.

Try to have one meat alternative daily.

dairy: 2 to 3 servings daily

You should have 2 to 3 daily servings of dairy. Dairy is a great source of calcium, protein, and the B vitamin riboflavin. Dairy also contains the magic ingredient for fullness: protein. In order to reap the fullness reward from protein-rich food, all you need to do is include a little bit with each meal. Low-fat dairy makes a great breakfast option. If you're tired of the same egg-white omelet or egg varieties, add a little milk, low-fat yogurt, and cheese to spice things up. This little trick turned things around for my client Nancy, a woman in her mid-forties, who was having the hardest time losing weight because she was always hungry. I suggested that she include a small amount of protein with each meal. A dairy fan, she included fat-free milk with cereal for breakfast and a low-fat yogurt in the afternoon for a snack. It made all the difference, and she dropped twenty pounds without the feeling of constant hunger.

Notice that frozen yogurt and ice cream aren't in the dairy section. You'll find them in Treats and Sweets. Three servings of ice cream has calcium, but it's not the healthful way to put dairy in your diet.

FAT-FREE, LOW-FAT, AND REDUCED-FAT DAIRY

Buttermilk, fat-free or low-fat, 1 cup	*1 baseball*
Cheese, parmesan, grated, 3–4 tbsp	*1½–2 walnuts*
Cottage cheese, fat-free or low-fat, ½ cup	*½ baseball*
Evaporated fat-free milk, ½ cup	*½ baseball*
Farmer cheese, fat-free or low-fat, ¼ cup	*1 golf ball*
Fat-free dry milk, ⅓ cup dry	*½ tennis ball*
Hard cheese, fat-free, part-skim, low-fat, or reduced-fat, 2 slices, 1½–2 oz	*2 CDs or 6–8 dice*

    (e.g., Jarlsberg, part-skim mozzarella, reduced-fat feta, reduced-fat swiss, 2 rounds of Laughing Cow Light or Mini Babybell Light)

Hoop cheese, ½ cup	*rounded handful*
Ice milk, 1 cup	*1 baseball*
Milk, fat-free or low-fat (1%), 1 cup or 8 fl oz	*1 baseball*
Pot cheese, ½ cup	*rounded handful*
Ricotta cheese, part-skim, ¼ cup	*1 golf ball*
Soy milk, calcium-fortified, fat-free or low-fat, 1 cup (not technically a dairy, but a good dairy substitute)	*1 baseball*
Yogurt, fat-free or low-fat, 1 cup	*1 container*

WHOLE-MILK DAIRY

Cheese, whole-milk varieties, 2 slices, 1½–2 oz	
(e.g., American, Brie, cheddar, Monterey Jack)	**2 CDs or 6–8 dice**
Evaporated whole milk, ½ cup	**½ baseball**
Goat's milk, 1 cup	**1 baseball**
Kefir, 1 cup	**1 baseball**
Whole milk, 1 cup or 8 fl oz	**1 baseball**
Yogurt, whole milk, 1 cup	**1 container**

Smart Bets: *fat-free, low-fat, and part-skim dairy products*

Limit: *whole-milk dairy*

Healthy Hints: *Include some dairy for breakfast or an afternoon snack; it's a great source of protein. It's much better to eat your dairy than to pop a pill.*

fat: 1 to 3 servings daily

Until recently, when bacon and cheese became "diet" food, people thought that fat was, well, fattening. Here's the deal. All fat has 9 calories a gram, compared to carbs and protein, which have 4 calories a gram. In other words, fat has more than twice as many calories as carbs.

So don't pile on the fats and oils, but don't eliminate them entirely—some are good for you and perform important nutritional tasks. You should have 1 to 3 servings daily. Choose fats sparingly, especially if you're trying to lose weight and need to limit calories. I know that 1 to 3 servings may *seem* like very little, especially in today's high-fat food world. But it could be worse. Could be teaspoons (a thumb tip) instead of tablespoons (½ walnut). And remember—there are 3 teaspoons in 1 tablespoon, so I am actually suggesting 3 to 9 teaspoons, which gives you plenty of room to decide how you want to spread it out during the day. The choice is yours.

• reality check—fat •

Fats have what I think of as concentrated calories—they really pack 'em in. For example, 1 cup of almonds is high in fat and has over 800 calories, whereas 1 cup of popcorn has no fat (if you skip the butter) and only 36 calories. The difference is even more pronounced when you compare fats and vegetables. You can eat 3 cups of cooked spinach for the same calories as 1 tablespoon of oil. You can pile on the veggies, feel full, and get some great nutrients all at once. Plus, you don't have to stare at a half-empty plate, an eater's nightmare.

Beware of hidden fats in butter, whole milk, full-fat cheese, margarine, oil, and salad dressing. A healthy "low-cal" salad can become a high-fat bonanza if you slather it in dressing, even if it is a healthy olive-oil based dressing! Use fats, such as salad dressing, to add a splash of flavor instead of making a meal of Brie. Remember, even if you classify foods as "good fats" or "healthy fats," they're still highly caloric. When Beth first came to see me, she was surprised to hear that she couldn't eat unlimited amounts of nuts, which she thought of as a "good fat." She said, "No wonder I'm not losing weight. I've been chomping on nuts all day." Just because a food is labeled "healthy" doesn't mean "more is better."

Also pay close attention to foods that are labeled low-fat. Low-fat foods still have calories, and the calories often come from added sugar. It's amazing how many foods carry the "low-fat" label, even a gargantuan muffin that tops out at a spectacular 800 calories. Low-fat does not necessarily mean low-calorie.

To reduce fat, choose low-fat methods of preparing food. Grill, bake, or broil fish and chicken. Fried foods, such as fried chicken and French fries, are loaded with fat. Remove the skin from your chicken before you eat it. Skin is pure fat. And when you have vegetables, steam them or microwave them. Very often you won't need any oil. Try squeezing on a lemon with a sprinkle of fresh herbs and spices to add some flavor. When you do sauté your vegetables, pay attention to the amount of oil you use. And the same goes for salads and veggies—the fat is in the dressing. I recommend using no more than 1 salad-dressing cap's worth of dressing. That's about 1 tablespoon (1 serving of fat).

It is easier when you prepare foods at home because you know how much oil goes into the dish. When you're dining out, look out for fat clues. The words "fried," "béarnaise," "dijonaise," and "alfredo" all mean high fat, as does "parmesan," which isn't just a dusting of cheese. It means fried and topped with cheese.

HEALTHY FATS

Avocado, ¼	
Nuts (peanuts, cashews, almonds, walnuts, pistachios, pecans), 1 oz (about ¼ cup)	*1 golf ball*
Oil (canola, corn, peanut, olive, safflower, sesame, soybean), 1 tbsp (3 tsp)	*½ shot glass*
Olives, 12–15	
Peanut butter and other nut butters, 1 tbsp	*½ walnut*
Salad dressing (olive-oil-based), 1 tbsp	*½ shot glass*
Salad dressing, reduced-fat, 2 tbsp	*1 shot glass*
Seeds (sesame, sunflower, pumpkin), 1 oz (about ¼ cup)	*1 golf ball*
Tahini paste, 1 tbsp	*½ walnut*

UNHEALTHY FATS

Butter, 1 tbsp	*½ walnut or 3 standard postal stamps*
Coconut, shredded, 3 tbsp	*1½ walnut*
Cream, half-and-half, 2 tbsp	*1 walnut*
Cream, 2 tbsp	*walnut*
Cream cheese, 1 tbsp	*½ walnut*
Margarine, 1 tbsp	*½ walnut*
Mayonnaise, 1 tbsp	*½ walnut*
Salad dressing (creamy), 1 tbsp	*½ shot glass*
Sour cream, 3 tbsp	*1½ walnuts*

Smart Bets: *healthy fats such as olive oil, canola oil, most vegetable oils, tahini, avocado, olives, nuts, nut butters, and seeds*

Limit: unhealthy fats such as butter, coconut oil, cream cheese, margarine, mayonnaise, and creamy salad dressing

Healthy hint: Every little bit counts.

treats and sweets:
0 to 2 servings daily

The tippy-top of the Portion Teller Pyramid is what I call "Treats and Sweets." It probably won't shock you to hear that sweets aren't part of a balanced diet. If you are not a treat eater, don't start now. Best to skip this if you can or have a small portion as a treat. These foods are filled with empty calories—lots of calories and very few, if any, nutrients. When it comes to Treats and Sweets, less is more.

But, boy, do they taste good, and indulgence is part of life. You might enjoy a nice glass of red wine with your meal, and I would never ask you to give that up. Eating should be a pleasure instead of a chore. But I want you to think about exactly when and how you want to treat yourself.

Before you snack, check your hunger level. Are you truly hungry or are you bored? Choose something you absolutely love as a snack and stick to it. You won't feel deprived and you won't overdo it.

GUIDELINES FOR TREATS AND SWEETS

1. Avoid your triggers—for some it's salty chips and for others it's sweets. Know yourself. If you know that you can't stop at a handful, don't even start. A handful of your favorite treat will not damage your weight-loss efforts, but eating an entire bag of something will.

2. Try not to have sweets daily. Make Fridays your splurge days. And don't eat tasteless cookies just because they're offered to you. Save up for what you really enjoy.

3. Skip sugar-sweetened beverages like soft drinks. It's best not to guzzle down those empty sugar calories—you won't feel like you've eaten. You're better off chewing. Plus, people end up eating junk with sodas, so they end up having two unhealthy snacks at once.

4. Fat-free doesn't mean sin-free. You'll gain weight if you eat too many of the fat-free varieties of cakes, cookies and ice creams. Portions always matter.

5. When you indulge at a restaurant, share dessert with a friend.

6. Remember that it's best to buy foods you can eat in units. A lollipop (a Tootsie Pop or a Blow Pop), a fudge pop, a frozen fruit bar, or a small bag of chips to share with a friend. If you are craving chocolate, buy one fun-size bar or two small peppermint patties instead of a regular-size candy bar.

7. Don't buy a pound of chocolate planning to save some for later. Let's be realistic. Leftovers don't work for most sugar lovers.

8. Don't buy big bags. Remember, some single-serve bags are still big.

9. Choose your evil and stick to it: a lollipop after dinner, ice cream once or twice a week.

10. Don't let "special" occasions be an excuse for cake, ice cream, and cupcakes. There are too many special occasions in life to allow yourself to indulge in all of them.

11. If you're trying to curb a sugar habit, start by substituting an extra serving of fruit for your sweet snack.

12. Don't let sweets become your "forbidden foods" that you crave because you can't have them. Change quantity and frequency using the tips above to work them into your food plan.

Alcoholic beverages	
5–6 oz wine	*6-oz yogurt container*
12 oz beer	*12-oz can*
Cakes and cookies, 1 oz	
Biscotti, 1	
Cookies, 2 (2 in)	*2 tea bags or size of 2 Oreos*
Cake, sliver, 1 oz	*CD case*
Cupcake, mini, 1 oz	*half-dollar size across*
Ginger Snaps, 2 (2 in)	*2 tea bags or size of 2 Oreos*
Pie, ⅓ cup	*golf ball, 4–5 forkfuls*
Candies and sweets,	
¼ cup unless indicated	*1 golf ball or 1 layer on your palm*
Chocolate	
1 bite-size, "fun-size," mini trick-or-treat-size bar	
2 small York Peppermint Patties	

4 Hershey's Kisses

M&M candies — *1 layer on your palm*

Cracker Jack, ½ cup — *½ baseball or 1 rounded handful*

Fruit roll-up, 1

Gummi bears — *1 layer on your palm*

Hard candy, 3

Jelly beans — *1 layer on your palm*

Licorice, 2 twists

Lollipop, 1 Tootsie Pop or Charms Blow Pop

Tootsie Rolls, 3 Midgies

Chips, ½ cup — *1 handful or ½ baseball*

(e.g., 15 corn chips, 10 potato chips, 15 soy crisps, 10 tortilla chips)

Energy/sports bar, 1 ounce — *1 Pria bar, ½ Balance bar, ½ Luna bar*

Fried foods

French fries, ½ cup — *1 handful or ½ baseball*

Frozen treats

Frozen fruit pop, 1

Fudgsicle pop, 1

Ice cream, ½ cup — *½ baseball*

Italian ice, ½ cup — *½ baseball*

Frozen yogurt, ½ cup — *½ baseball*

Low-fat or fat-free ice cream, ½ cup — *½ baseball*

Sorbet, ½ cup — *½ baseball*

Gravies and sauces, 2 tbsp — *1 walnut in a shell*

Soft drinks, sugar-sweetened beverages, 8 oz — *small Styrofoam cup or 8-oz yogurt container*

Sugar, honey, jelly, maple syrup, 2 tbsp — *1 walnut in a shell*

Lesser Evils:

Baked potato and tortilla chips: Baked Lays potato chips, Baked Doritos

Barry's French Twists

Fortune cookie

Frozen fruit pop (noncreamy varieties such as strawberry, raspberry, lemon, lime)

Jell-O
Low-fat or fat-free frozen yogurt or dietary dessert (TCBY, Tasti-D-Lite,
    Colombo)
Popsicle
"The Skinny Cow" Silhouette fudge bar, flying saucer, or ice cream sundae
Soy Crisps
Sorbet (noncreamy varieties such as mixed berry, raspberry, lemon)

Consider these suggested snacks: fresh fruit, low-fat yogurt, a piece of string cheese, baby carrots, celery and peppers with hummus or salsa, V8 juice, vegetable soup, popcorn, a homemade smoothie, a rice cake and peanut butter, a whole-grain crisp bread (Kavli, Ryvita, or Finn Crisp) with a slice of low-fat cheese, a handful of nuts, a frozen banana with peanut butter, frozen melon cubes, a baked apple with 1 teaspoon of brown sugar and a dash of cinnamon.

• reality check—salt •

Good old table salt is the common name for sodium chloride, which contains 40 percent sodium. Sodium is found in lots of foods. We do need some salt in our diet, but it's not a good idea to overdo it. Anyone who is watching his weight needs to be on the lookout for "water weight" gain, which is partly due to salt consumption.

The more a food is processed, the more sodium it usually contains. Some common foods that contain sodium are: table salt, bouillon cubes, baking soda, soy sauce, horseradish, MSG, pickles, sauerkraut, processed meats and cheeses, frozen dinners, packaged mixes, and salted snacks such as chips, nuts, and pretzels, and canned soups. Foods described as cured, pickled, corned, or smoked are high in sodium. To cut back and shake the salt habit, remember: The less processed the food, the less sodium it contains. Try to include fresh or frozen rather than canned veggies. Limit other processed meats and cheeses and frozen meals. Keep the salt shaker in the cabinet instead of out on the kitchen table. Flavor foods with spices and herbs. Go easy on condiments such as mustard, ketchup, and soy sauce. A shake, sprinkle, or taste here and there adds up quickly!

water

Drink 64 ounces water (eight 8-ounce glasses): water, seltzer, herbal tea

exercise: 30 minutes, 3 to 4 times a week

Aim for a minimum of 30 minutes of aerobic exercise (brisk walking, swimming, hiking, power yoga, biking, or jogging) at least three to four times a week along with a short period of resistance or weight-bearing exercise. Try to find something you like, so it won't feel like a chore. There are two parts to the weight-loss equation: Eat less + move more!

If you have a hard time working exercise into your schedule, opt for "lifestyle exercise." If you usually cook dinner for your family, you can do 20 or 30 canned-food arm curls, for example. Do leg lifts while you chat on the phone. Mow your own lawn. Try to incorporate small amounts of exercise into your daily routine; take the stairs instead of elevators or escalators, park your car a few blocks away and walk, get off the bus one stop before your destination, or go for a walk at lunchtime. A few changes like these add up over the course of the day.

You don't have to belong to a fancy gym to incorporate exercise into your life. If you don't exercise at all, start small. Adding even two rounds of fifteen-minute exercise is progress. Work your way up to thirty minutes three times per week. Brisk walking is great. Just move more! Pick exercises you enjoy and find fun.

If you can manage more exercise, try for five days per week, and gradually increase your workout time to forty-five minutes. You can always do stretching, floor exercises, and deep knee-bends while watching TV. If you have some reading to do, hop on the StairMaster or stationary bike with your book or magazine.

Give yoga a shot. It isn't just for flower children anymore. It helps you become more flexible, increases strength, improves balance, and relieves stress. And you feel rejuvenated afterward.

• get smart! •

- Cut out food from one food group, and you usually end up eating too much from another food group.
- Nobody ever got fat eating too many carrots.
- Follow the rainbow: Choose an assortment of colorful fruits and veggies. The more colorful your diet, the more antioxidants and phytonutrients you're getting (that is, the healthier your diet).
- The best dose of health comes from healthy foods, not from pills.
- No-fat and low-fat foods still contain calories.
- "Diet food" may seem enticing, but it never helped us lose weight. There's more of it on the market than ever before, but we're fatter than ever. The scale speaks for itself.
- "Energy" is the scientific term for calories, so "energy bars" also can be called "calorie bars." They're no miracle food, nor are they diet food. Have them as a treat, not as a daily snack, especially if you're trying to lose weight.
- Low-carb cakes, cookies, and beer are no "cake walk" or miracle cure.
- Fat hides calories. When you trim it from your diet, you cut calories.
- A little lean protein at each meal goes a long way to making you feel full.
- Make healthy eating a habit, not a diet.
- And finally: If you want to lose weight, you have to cut back on how much you eat. There's no getting around it.

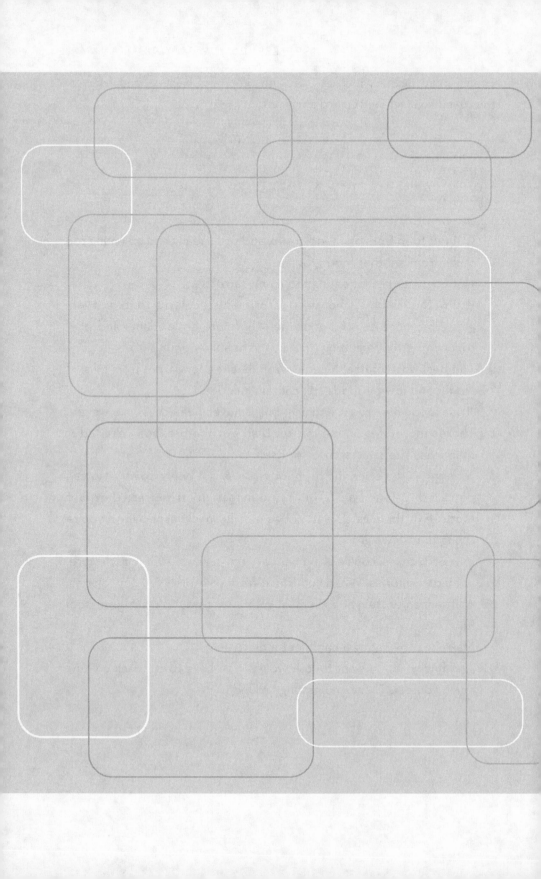

size matters

When asked if I wanted my pizza cut into
four or eight slices, I replied: Four.
I don't think I can eat eight.
• YOGI BERRA

making smartsize substitutions

et's talk about what you normally have for breakfast. There's a good chance that your breakfast includes something starchy. We love our breads and grains, especially in the morning: muffins of all kinds, bagels, English muffins, croissants, toast, and cereals. Grains can be a great way to start the day, but *what* kind of grain you choose and *how much* of it makes a big difference when it comes to managing your weight. If you're like many people, you probably assume that one of these starchy items isn't much different from another—a bagel is about the same as an English muffin or two pieces of toast. But now you know that's wrong.

Clearly, not all bagels are equal. The shocking truth is that today's bagel translates into 2½ English muffins or 5 slices of bread, which is almost half a loaf. That means that you could eat 5 slices of bread for the same amount of calories as your breakfast bagel. Hold a bagel in one hand. Now hold a slice of bread in your other hand. Feel their weights, balancing them up and down. Doesn't the bagel weigh more than the slice of bread? In fact, doesn't it weigh a lot more? It should: It's five times as heavy.

This difference in size translates into a big difference in servings. Five times the size, in the case of the bagel/bread comparison, means five times the servings. When we're talking about a muffin that weighs as much as a softball, it can easily reach 800 calories, up from 150 calories in the not-so-distant past. Typical portions are two to five times the size they were in the 1970s, translating into two to five times the calories. Even the dough in your lunchtime pizza slice now translates to three slices of bread, and that doesn't include the cheese, sauce, and toppings. Dealing with such a wide range of calories means a world of difference when it comes to weight gain or loss. Understanding today's portion sizes is crucial. It is the key to smartsizing and managing your weight.

PORTION CHECK: HOW MANY SERVINGS ARE YOU EATING?

1 cup cooked rice	=	1 baseball	=	2 grain servings
1 6-oz salmon steak (cooked)	=	2 decks of cards	=	2 meat servings
1 9-oz steak (cooked)	=	3 decks of cards	=	3 meat servings
1 sweet potato	=	1 computer mouse	=	2 grain/starchy vegetable servings

So how do you make substitutions? Take our favorite bagel. If you're in the mood for some grains, you could go ahead and eat that bagel, or you could consult the "Size Matters: Common Foods and Their Equivalents" section on page 81 and see that, for a similar calorie and nutrient profile, you could have 10 rice cakes, 15 cups of popcorn, or 120 oyster crackers. You probably will be shocked to learn that an average bran muffin (not the biggest around) equals 6½ waffles. You probably wouldn't dream of eating that many waffles, but wouldn't think twice about having a bran muffin, even if it's big. And, just because it is called a "bran" muffin, it is not necessarily health food. The same can be said for juice. Many people guzzle a pint of orange juice, but would never have the equivalent—3 oranges, 6 tangerines, or 75 grapes—in one sitting. There is something very psychologically comforting about saying "I only ate one." Who wouldn't feel like a glutton if they ate 6½ waffles or 120 mini pretzels all at once? But the comfort of "I only ate one" is very deceptive, especially when that "one" is giant size.

Now you have the tools to make choices. Look at the "Size Matters" section to see your favorite foods and what foods are roughly equivalent to them. For example, a bagel = 2½ English muffins = 5 slices of bread = 10 rice cakes = 15 cups popcorn, and so on. Once you learn this, you can reconsider how you want to use those grain servings. There are many options, and every one

• portion patrol •

Help! I'm scared that if I eat any bread I won't be able to lose weight.

If you have bread phobia, eat starchy vegetables and brown rice instead of bread. When you do eat bread, choose whole grains such as 100 percent whole wheat. I've seen countless people lose weight on 4 starches per day. The key is to choose wisely! And, remember, a bagel is not 1 to 2 servings. It is more like 5. When you cut out bread completely, you do lose weight quickly, for two reasons:

1. You often end up eating less food.

2. When you drastically reduce carbs, you lose lots of water weight.

The problem is that you probably cannot sustain this type of diet over the long haul. It's too hard to feel satisfied. And as soon as you introduce starches, you'll just gain back the water weight you lost.

is acceptable. You can eat half a bagel or you can eat the whole bagel, but scoop out the center if you're not attached to it. Or maybe you'd rather have that big ole bagel for breakfast and blow all your grains before 10 A.M., but be sure to count it as 5 grain servings. Or, maybe you want to skip the bagel, which you can do without, have cereal or an English muffin, and opt for some rice with dinner. It's your choice. You don't have to cut out all starch, or even all bagels from your diet. Starches and breads aren't fattening. Often they're just too big. But you can make comfortable substitutions that bring your portions down to size. One slice of bread or a pita pocket will not make you fat. And keep in mind the Smart Bets—whole grains are always better than white-bread products.

If you can make simple substitutions within the same food groups—an orange instead of a pint of orange juice—you'll know that you're saving calories. In the case of the orange, you're having almost one-third the calories of the juice. Even though I'm telling you that you'll save calories by making these substitutions, again, this program is not about *counting* calories. If you learn how big the foods you eat are and how they compare to other foods, you can cut down in calories without actually counting them. Take a look at the comparisons beginning on page 81. You don't have to know how many calories are in any of the foods. All you have to know is that by choosing your foods wisely, you've just saved a load of calories before 10 A.M. Once you learn the food equivalents, you can plan ahead, and decide what foods you can't live without and where you can cut calories without feeling deprived.

It's all about smartsizing. Just the simple switch from a bagel to an English muffin—and nothing else—on a daily basis saves you at least 200 calories a day, which translates into a weight loss of twenty pounds a year. Even just leaving a bit on your plate, and not finishing your pizza slice, bagel, or muffin, can save you 100 calories, translating into a ten-pound weight loss over a year. Think about how easily you could make this kind of switch without any feeling of loss or deprivation. The trick to not being hungry is to include some protein with your grain such as a slice of Jarlsburg cheese with tomato or some cottage cheese or an egg. Now you can have some of the grains you love for breakfast—but an English muffin instead of a blueberry muffin—and start the day with a satisfied smile, all the while losing weight over the year. These small changes can make the difference between fitting into your "skinny" jeans or not, which is what so many of us struggle with on a daily basis. The comparisons in "Size Matters" (page 81), and those that you design for yourself with the help of Appendix D train your eye and memory so that you never look at a bagel or a muffin in the same way again. Instead of seeing a bagel, you just may see your new favorite breakfast, your painless new way to reduce how much you eat.

• reality check •

I've mentioned that a bagel is the equivalent of 5 slices of bread. This doesn't mean you should go out and eat 5 slices of bread instead of a bagel. The comparisons are trying to make a point. If a bran muffin is equivalent to eating 6½ waffles, maybe you'll think twice about eating the bran muffin. You could eat 3 waffles and feel comparatively virtuous.

serving size substitutions

To practice portion awareness in your daily life, you must known three things:

1. The different food groups
2. How to choose the right amount from each group
3. The key to smartsizing: how to make trade-offs, or substitutions, within each group

A standard serving size is meaningful only if it works as a comparison and helps you understand the relative nutritional worth, or, where possible, caloric worth, of your food. Within the food groups, especially the grain group, the serving size I give you for each item has a similar calorie count to all the other items. A 1-ounce serving of whole-grain bread, crackers, and tortillas have a similar nutrient and calorie profile. In the dairy group, many of the choices have a similar amount of calcium, but whole-milk dairy clearly contains more calories than the low-fat dairy products. Foods in the meat group have similar amounts of protein but not necessarily the same calorie counts. The calories diverge more widely in the meat group because of the varying fat content of meat, poultry, fish, and meat alternatives. A serving of steak, for example, is usually very fatty and has many more calories than a serving of canned tuna; however, the protein content is roughly equivalent.

Despite some of these caloric deviations, feel free to pick and choose widely within each group, trading off one food for another without counting calories. Take a look at the grain group: 1 piece of bread is 1 serving. For a similar calorie count, you can substitute it for anything else on the grains/starch list: ½ cup (½ baseball) of cooked rice or pasta, 1 cup (1 baseball) of cereal flakes, 3 cups (3 baseballs) of popcorn, and so on. The underlying reason you lose weight, in any weight-loss program is because you cut back on calories. If you want to be sure that you are getting the least amount of calories for the most nutrients, as well as the most fiber, always pick the Smart Bets from each food category, as discussed in the previous chapter.

Now that you have a greater understanding of serving sizes under your belt, you've got everything you need to guide your daily food choices. Don't forget—all of the visuals provided make comparisons within the same food group. I never compare popcorn to chicken breast. That trade-off may have the exact same calories, but that's not what's most important. Since our ultimate goal is health and well-being (which means maintaining a healthy weight), using calorie comparisons alone just doesn't make sense. Trade-offs within the same food group ensure that you get all the nutrients you need for a well-balanced diet.

PORTION TELLER AWARENESS EQUATION

Know the food groups + Know the Smart Bets from each food group + Know the number of servings per day per food group + Know the standard serving size of each food. Knowledge is portion power.

size matters: common foods and their equivalents*

Bagel (5 ounces) = 5 grain servings

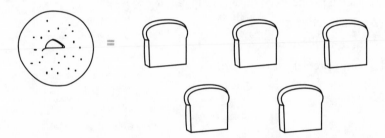

1 cup (1 baseball) cereal flakes + 2 slices bread + 1 cup (1 baseball) rice or

2½ English muffins or

2½ cups (2½ baseballs) rice or

2½ baked potatoes (each the size of a computer mouse) or

5 slices bread or

10 cups (10 baseballs) puffed wheat cereal or

10 rice cakes or

15 cups (15 baseballs) popcorn or

120 oyster crackers

*Disclaimer: The foods on the next several pages aren't exactly alike nutritionally or calorically. Few foods are exactly equal, but these food group equivalents will help you make better choices.

Street (soft) pretzel
(6 ounces) = 6 grain servings

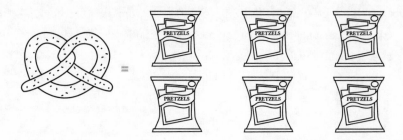

1 cup (1 baseball) Cheerios + 1 (4-inch) pita the diameter of a CD + 3
   cups (3 baseballs) popcorn + 1 cup (1 baseball) rice or couscous + 2
   pretzel rods or

6 1-ounce bags pretzels or

6 1-ounce pretzels (Bavarian, Baldies) or

12 pretzel rods or

54 three-ring pretzels or

120 mini pretzels

Bran muffin (6.5 ounces) = 6 ½ grain servings

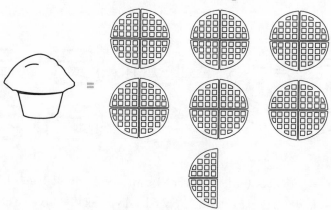

4 cups (4 baseballs) puffed wheat + 2 slices bread + 1 cup (1 baseball) cooked pasta + 1½ cups (1½ baseballs) popcorn or

6½ cups (6½ baseballs) bran flakes or

6½ waffles or

65 mini flavored rice cakes or

52 animal crackers

Pasta entrée in a restaurant (3 cups pasta) = 6 grain servings

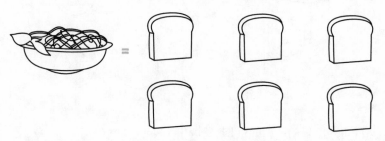

1 cup (1 baseball) bran flakes + 2 slices bread + 1 cup (1 baseball) rice or couscous + 3 cups (3 baseballs) popcorn or

3 cups (3 baseballs) rice or

6 slices bread or

18 cups (18 baseballs) popcorn

Steak at a steakhouse
(24-ounce precooked yields approximately
18 ounces cooked) = 6 meat servings

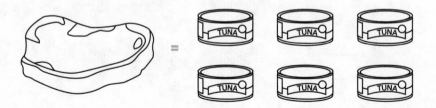

3 eggs + 3 ounces (1 deck of cards) turkey + 1 cup (1 baseball) lentils +
6 ounces (2 decks of cards) cooked sirloin steak + 3-ounce can tuna or
3 pieces cooked salmon, 6 ounces each (each the size of 2 decks of cards) or
Six 3-ounce cans tuna or
18 eggs

Pint orange juice (16 fluid ounces) =
almost 3 fruit servings

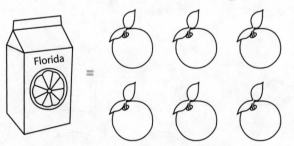

1 orange+ 2 kiwi+ 1 cup (1 baseball) blueberries or
2½–3 cups (2½–3 baseballs) cantaloupes or
2½–3 cups (2½–3 baseballs) mixed berries or
2½–3 cups (2½–3 baseballs) grapes (approx 75–90 grapes) or
3 oranges or
6 tangerines

To see smartsizing in action, let me give you two real-life examples based on the preferences of two of my clients. Jessie and Barbara like different foods and have different eating habits, so I tailored a program that allows them to have what they like, to make their own choices, as long as their food groups are balanced throughout the day.

Jessie loves pasta and would prefer to save up her grains so that she can have a bowl of pasta for dinner at a restaurant. Barbara likes to have her grains spread out throughout the day, including a little at each meal. Both women are aiming to eat only 5 grains a day since they are trying to lose weight and want to be fairly strict about their intake.

Let's look at Jessie: Since a standard serving of pasta is ½ cup cooked (½ baseball), she can have up to 2½ cups cooked (2½ baeballs) at dinner (5 grain servings per day x ½ baseball or ½ cup, which is the standard serving size). You know that a pasta entrée at a restaurant averages about 3 cups cooked (3 baseballs), so to eat her goal of 2½ cups, Jessie should leave a little on her plate. Or she can choose an appetizer portion, which is usually 1½ cups cooked (1½ baseballs), or 3 servings, and have a thick slice of bread along with dinner to sop up the tomato sauce or a sandwich on whole-wheat bread at lunch. It's not ideal to eat pasta as an entrée on a daily basis because it is a white-flour product and lacks fiber. When she has pasta, Jessie makes sure to eat plenty of veggies. She also eats whole-wheat pasta when possible (and eats some whole grains on the days that it's not possible). Rather than banning a pasta entrée entirely, Jessie has it once a week, which helps her stick with her program on other days. Being "allowed" to eat foods you love makes a huge difference in how successful you will be in sticking to a weight-loss program.

Now on to Barbara: she can do without pasta altogether but likes to get her grains throughout the day. She has 1 cup (1 baseball) of Cheerios for breakfast (1 grain), 2 pieces of bread on a sandwich at lunch (2 grains), and 1 cup (1 baseball) of rice with her Chinese dinner (2 grains). If she cuts back on the rice at dinner to ½ cup (½ baseball), she can even have an evening snack of 8 animal crackers (1 grain), which she loves.

Once you have an idea of exactly how big a serving size is, you can pick and choose anything from the list.

Jessie's Choice

2½ cups (2½ baseballs)
    pasta

Barbara's Choice

1 cup (1 baseball) cereal + 2 slices bread +
    1 cup baseball rice
1 cup (1 baseball) cereal + 2 slices bread +
    ½ cup (½ baseball) rice + 8 animal
    crackers

All choices equal 5 grain servings a day.

Other Examples

Sue likes to save her meat for a dinner out, whereas Michele wants to spread out her meats during the day, eating a bit for lunch, snacks, and dinner. Let's see how that plays out.

Sue's Choice

8 ounces chicken or
    fish (approximately
    3 decks of cards
    worth)

Michele's Choice

3 oz (1 deck of cards of turkey) +
    1 cup (1 baseball) of beans or bean
    soup + 3 oz (1 deck of cards) fish

Both choices equal roughly 3 meat servings a day.

Mike wants to grab an occasional pint of juice in the morning on the way to his meeting, whereas Steven wants to spread out his fruit snacks during the day.

Mike's Choice

Pint orange juice

Steven's Choice

1 cup (1 baseball) berries + 1 baseball-sized
    apple + ½ grapefruit

Both choices equal 3 fruit servings a day.

Remember, it is all about choice.

• reality check— weight vs. volume •

Did you know that puffed wheat is a lot lighter than any granola? How's this for confusing: 1 ounce cold cereal equals about 2 cups (2 baseballs) puffed wheat, or 1 cup (1 baseball) flakes, or ¼ cup (1 golf ball) granola. It's impossible to memorize all the different weights, especially when weight is not commonly used to describe cereal.

Another common cereal measuring mistake is the assumption that 1 cup equals 8 ounces for all foods. That equation applies only to liquids. That's why I use cups as serving sizes for cold cereal—the same unit I use for rice, pasta, and cooked cereals—in addition to giving you the weight. I don't want you to run into the same problem as Michele, who carried around a huge plastic sack of cereal as a snack, thinking that 1 cup equaled 8 ounces! Michele measured out 8 ounces as her portion. She didn't understand that 8 ounces of cereal is actually 8 cups. Imagine 8 baseballs! Then why is a ½ baseball the visual for one serving of pasta and for one serving of tomato sauce even though one is a solid and one a liquid? For foods such as pasta, rice, and tomato sauce, most people think about the amount they eat in volume measures such as cups. The visuals I provide are volume measures, so they work for liquids and solids. Where necessary, I've already taken the density of foods into account so you don't have to.

SHARPEN YOUR VISUAL SKILLS

- Copy the visuals from Chapter 2 and put them on your fridge. Or, if you prefer draw an outline of your own hand on a sheet of paper and put it on the fridge, making a note of what the measurements are (1 thumb = teaspoon, 1 finger = 1 ounce cheese, etc.).

- If you're feeling unsure about your visual skills and estimating your portions, keep a CD, a deck of cards, a walnut in the shell, a baseball, a golf ball, a shot glass, a postal stamp, and a plastic water bottle cap around the house. Put them in the bowl you used to keep your unlimited supply of candy or nuts in, and look at them occasionally.

• portion patrol•

Help! I overate today. Does that mean that I totally blew my food plan?

Here's your mantra: *If I eat more today, there is always tomorrow.*

You don't want to make this a daily mantra, but if you do overindulge on occasion, don't consider yourself a failure. Get right back on track. If you overate starches today, eat fewer starches tomorrow. But don't starve yourself, and *do not* skip meals. And be sure to include some protein at each meal.

restaurant survival guide: how do restaurant portions stack up?

Do you love going out to dinner? Who doesn't? Don't stop dining out—doing so is not only impractical, it's downright boring. You don't have to quit having fun to maintain a healthy weight. It doesn't matter how much the restaurant serves you; what matters is how much you actually eat! You do need to be careful and make educated choices. You are in control. Practice defensive dining!

Of course, some restaurants serve larger portions than others, but this guide will help you approximate.

RESTAURANT SURVIVAL GUIDE

FOOD	PORTION SIZE	VISUAL	SERVINGS PER FOOD GROUP
Restaurant			
Hamburger patty	4–6 oz cooked	1–2 decks of cards	1½–2 meat
Bun	3 oz	1 baseball	3 grain
Fries	2 cups	2 baseballs	4 high-fat treats
Chicken, fish, or beef entrée	6–9 oz cooked	2–3 decks of cards	2–3 meat
Cooked vegetable, side dish	1 cup	1 baseball	2 vegetable
Rice, side dish	1 cup	1 baseball	2 grain
Tossed salad with dressing			
Salad	2–3 cups	2–3 baseballs	2–3 vegetable

FOOD	PORTION SIZE	VISUAL	SERVINGS PER FOOD GROUP
Dressing (salad dressing ladle)	3-4 Tbsp (¼ cup)	1 golf ball	3-4 fat
Soda	16 fl oz and up		2+ treats: lots of sugar

Steakhouse

Steak	7 + oz cooked	2+ decks of cards	2 + meat
Baked potato, side order	8-16 oz (1 lb)		2-4 grain/starchy vegetable
Cooked vegetable, side order	1-2 cups	1-2 baseballs	2-4 vegetable
Tossed salad with dressing			
Salad	2-3 cups	2-3 baseballs	2-3 vegetable
Dressing (salad dressing ladle)	3-4 Tbsp (¼ cup)	1 golf ball	3-4 fat
Dressing on side	use 1 Tbsp	½ shot glass	1 fat

Italian

Pasta entrée	3 cups pasta	3 baseballs	6 grain
Pasta appetizer	1½ cups pasta	1½ baseballs	3 grain
Garlic bread, 1 piece	2 oz	bar of soap	2 grain
Chicken, fish, or beef entrée	6-8 oz cooked	2-3 decks of cards	2-3 meat
Tossed salad with dressing			
Salad	2 cups	2 baseballs	2 vegetable
Salad dressing	3-4 Tbsp (¼ cup)	1 golf ball	3-4 fat

FOOD	PORTION SIZE	VISUAL	SERVINGS PER FOOD GROUP
Chinese			
Chicken and vegetables	**3-4 cups**	**3-4 baseballs**	
vegetables	**2-3 cups**	**2-3 baseballs**	**4-6 vegetable**
chicken	**6-8 oz**	**2-3 decks of cards**	**2-3 meat**
Sauce, varies	**4 Tbsp**	**about 2 walnuts**	**3-5 fat**
Sauce on side	**1 Tbsp**	**½ walnut**	**1 fat**
Rice, steamed, side order			
eat in	**1 cup**	**1 baseball**	**2 grain**
takeout/order in, pint-size	**2 cups**	**2 baseballs**	**4 grain**
Steamed vegetable dumplings	**2 large dumplings**		**1 grain, small amount vegetable**
Japanese			
Sushi, 1 roll (6 pieces)			
rice	**½-1 cup**	**½-1 baseball**	**1-2 grain**
Fish—varies by type of roll	**2-3 oz**	**deck of cards**	**1 meat**
Assorted vegetables	**½ cup**	**½ baseball**	**1 vegetable**
Avocado			**½ fat**
Note: "spicy" rolls contain mayonnaise		½ walnut	1 fat
Chicken, fish, beef, grilled or teriyaki	**6-8 oz cooked**	**2-3 decks of cards**	**2-3 meat**

FOOD	PORTION SIZE	VISUAL	SERVINGS PER FOOD GROUP
Rice, side order	1 cup	1 baseball	2 grain
Cooked vegetable	½–1 cup	½–1 baseball	1–2 vegetable

Mexican
Burrito

Tortilla	2 oz	2 CD cases	2 grain
Rice	up to ½ cup	½ baseball	1 grain
Beans	up to ½ cup	½ baseball	1 grain/starchy vegetable
Cheese	1–2 oz	4–8 dice	1 dairy
Salad	½ cup	½ baseball	½ vegetable
Guacamole	2–4 Tbsp	1–2 walnuts	1 fat
Sour cream	2–3 Tbsp	1–1½ walnuts	1 fat

Deli
Sandwich

Traditional

Sliced bread	2 slices	2 CD cases	2 grain
Meat filling	5–8 oz	5–8 CDs	2–3 meat (1 day's worth)
Cheese (optional)	1–2 oz	1–2 CDs	1 dairy
Lettuce/ tomato	varies		small amount of vegetable

Hero/Submarine sandwich

Small sub	6 inch	half a ruler	2½ grain
Ft.-long sub	12 inch	1 ruler	5 grain
Meat filling	3–7 oz*	3–7 CDs	1–2½ meat
Cheese	1–2 oz	1–2 CDs	1 dairy
Lettuce/ tomato	varies		vegetable

*Small subs contain about 3 ounces meat filling. Large subs contain more.

FOOD	PORTION SIZE	VISUAL	SERVINGS PER FOOD GROUP
Coffee House			
12-oz tall latte or cappuccino	*12 fl oz*	*1 soda can*	*1 dairy*
20-oz venti latte or cappuccino	*20 fl oz*	*1 ¾ soda cans*	*2 dairy*
Other			
Fruit smoothie	*16–24 fl oz*	*1½–2 soda cans*	*3–4 fruit*
Pizza slice (individual)	*7–8 oz*		*3–4 grain* *1–2 dairy* *1 vegetable* *some added fat*
Fruit juice	*16 fl oz*	*1 pint*	*almost 3 fruit*

visuals for typical marketplace portions

Cooked steak in a standard American restaurant = 8.1 ounces =

 2¾ decks of cards (more than an entire day's worth of meat)

Cooked steak in a steakhouse = 18 ounces =

 6 decks of cards or

6 palms of your hand (3 days' worth of meat)

Pasta entrée = 3 cups =

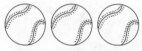

3 baseballs or

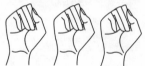

3 tight fists (entire day's worth of grains)

Hot pretzel = 6 ounces = 6 CD cases

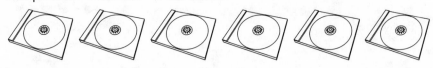

Pint OJ = 16 fl ounces =

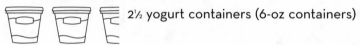

2½ yogurt containers (6-oz containers)

Pizza slice =

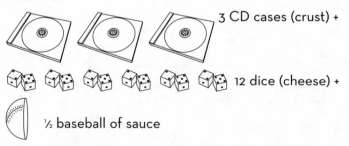

3 CD cases (crust) +

12 dice (cheese) +

½ baseball of sauce

Side dish of rice at a Chinese or Japanese restaurant = 1 cup =

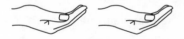 1 baseball or 1 fist or

 2 handfuls

Side of rice when ordering in Chinese food = 1 pint = 2 cups rice =

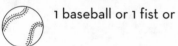 2 baseballs

Turkey sandwich (meat only) = 6 ounces =

 2 palms of your hand

Piece of bread from a bread basket = 2–3 ounces =

 2–3 CD cases

• reality check—france •

Smaller portions in France than in the U.S. help explain the "French Paradox" according to researchers at University of Pennsylvania and CNRS in Paris:

- Although the French eat more fat than Americans, they eat less than Americans.

- Portion sizes in American eating establishments are 25 percent larger than they are in Parisian eating establishments.

- Meals served in Chinese restaurants in Philadelphia are 72 percent heftier than those served in Chinese restaurants in Paris.

- Fourteen out of 17 single-serve items are larger in American supermarkets than in Parisian supermarkets. For example, a single-serve soft drink available in an American supermarket is 52 percent larger than a soft drink available in a Parisian supermarket.

- Portion size is mentioned more frequently (9.3 percent) in American restaurant reviews such as *Zagat* than in its Parisian counterpart (3.5 percent).

- French recipe portions are smaller than American recipe portions.

- Even though the French eat less, they spend more time eating. In a Parisian McDonald's, customers averaged 22.2 minutes at a table, compared with 14.4 minutes at an American McDonald's. The lesson: Eat more slowly.

your portion personality

What kind of sandwich isn't fattening?
Half a sandwich.
* CONVERSATION BETWEEN GANGSTERS IN
THE MOVIE *ANALYZE THIS*

he *Portion Teller* doesn't tell you what you can and can't eat, and there is no such thing as a "right" portion. A healthy food plan is all about balance. But just because there are no "off limits" foods doesn't mean you can eat whatever you want, whenever you want. Instead, you can eat what you want, when you want, as long as you balance your portions throughout the day and eat a healthy mix of foods from each of the food groups. By now you've started to develop portion-size awareness and nutrition awareness. Now we need to work on self-awareness so that you can tailor an eating plan that works for you and you alone.

The first step is to assess your food personality. Just the mere mention of "food" and "eating" brings up many personal memories, emotions, and powerful images. It's impossible to wipe out a lifetime of feelings and biases about food with an imposed eating plan; that's why I work *with* you and your habits instead of *against* you.

the portion checkup

Let's take a portion checkup. It's like when you go to a doctor and want to know what's wrong with you. Before the doctor can begin to diagnose you, she needs to determine your overall health, and usually starts with questions about your habits, a physical exam, and blood work. Well, this is the same thing. I'm going to ask you to keep a daily Portion Teller Diary. I promise you won't be tied to it forever, but there's no better way to take an "X-ray" of your diet, to get an overview of your eating habits. You can't address problems in your diet if you don't have a sense of what you usually eat, when you eat, and how much you eat. You will find a blank Portion Teller Diary in Appendix B. I suggest you make copies of those pages and place them in a binder or notebook to fill out on a daily basis. Using the Portion Teller Diary is the easiest and fastest way to figure out your food habits, what foods cause problems for you, and whether you eat out of boredom or stress. Once you understand your relationship with food, you can begin to introduce small, simple changes that will make a big difference over the long run.

For the first week, you're just going to use the diary to understand your habits. Do your best to record the portions and food groups for everything you eat. That's all. Ease yourself into it. It's an evaluation period. Keeping a food diary reveals eating patterns you may not have been aware of. Recognizing these patterns helps you develop effective strategies to lose weight. You also become more aware of what and how much you're eating. When you know you're going to write down every nibble, you might start to have second thoughts: Do I really need this? Don't hesitate to make some smartsize substitutions.

WATCH THE POUNDS DISAPPEAR

The goals of changing the way you eat are to be healthier and, for most of us, to drop unwanted pounds. Watching those pounds evaporate can be pretty inspiring, so sometimes it's fun to do a little more than rely on the scale. If you're exercising more and building muscle, the scale doesn't tell the whole story.

- Sometimes people lose weight and still think of themselves as fat. It helps actually to see the difference. Ask a friend to take "before" and "after" pictures of you.

- Pick a pair of skinny pants that you want to fit into again. Don't pick pants from your fifth-grade class photo, though. Be reasonable! Try them on once a week to see yourself getting closer to your goal.

- Use a measuring tape to measure the inches around your waist, chest, hips (at the widest part), and thighs. Write the measurements down and track the changes weekly.

- Don't weigh yourself several times a day or even every day. Cut back to once a week if you absolutely need the scale to measure your progress.

eight simple steps

Time for a bite of reality. Let's walk through the Portion Teller Diary and learn how to enter your daily diet information.

1. *Write down everything you eat.* Include all tastes, sips, and little bites that you have throughout the day. They can add up, and when you write them down, you are forced to acknowledge that you ate them—even if you nibble while standing in front of the fridge, stopping by the office kitchen, or running to catch the bus. Also include how you prepared your meals—baked, broiled, fried, and so on.

2. *Record your portion.* Write down exactly how much you ate. You can be as strict as you want here; if you prefer to measure your food in the beginning, that's okay. But try using the visuals. For example, 1 cup of Cheerios is the size of a tight fist or a baseball. The 3-ounce turkey breast is the size of your palm or a deck of cards. The tablespoonful of peanut butter is the size of three thumb tips or ½ a walnut.

3. *Place the food you ate in the right food group.* If you had a glass of milk, enter it into the dairy group. If you had some oatmeal, put it in the grain group. If you have any questions about the food groups, refer to Chapter 3 and Appendix D.

4. *Break the portion you ate into standard serving sizes.* Consult the serving size chart in Appendix D and apply it to your portion. For example, if you had 1 cup (1 baseball) of cooked rice or couscous, count it as 2 grain servings. If you had a bagel, count it as 5 grain servings. A muffin is at least 6 grain servings. A pasta entrée at a restaurant is 6 grain servings. A 6-ounce salmon fillet (2 decks of cards) is 2 meat servings.

5. *Tally up the servings from each food group for the day.* Count up how many servings you had from each food group.

6. *Cross off the appropriate serving graphic in the diary.* If you figured out that you had 2 grain servings, cross off 2 grain graphics on the diary to show that you've used up 2 of your daily servings. Do this for everything you eat during the day.

7. *Don't forget to include water.*

8. *Write down what kind of exercise you do and for how long.*

Portion Teller Diary

FOOD (INCLUDE METHOD OF PREPARATION)	YOUR PORTION	FOOD GROUP	NUMBER OF SERVINGS
BREAKFAST:			
LUNCH:			
SNACK:			
DINNER:			

FOOD	YOUR PORTION	FOOD GROUP	NUMBER OF SERVINGS
(INCLUDE METHOD OF PREPARATION)			

SNACK:

FRUITS:

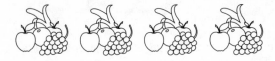

VEGETABLES:

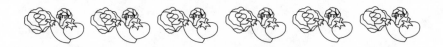

GRAINS AND STARCHY VEGETABLES:

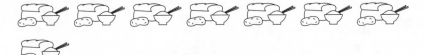

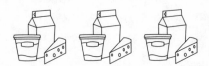

DAIRY:

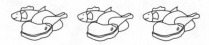

FISH, POULTRY, MEATS, AND MEAT ALTERNATIVES:

FATS:

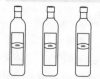

TREATS AND SWEETS:

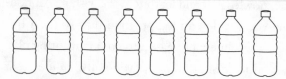

WATER:

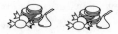

EXERCISE:

PORTION TELLER PROGRESS:

your portion personality

Now that you're keeping your Portion Teller Diary, let's take a closer look at your Portion Personality. Eating isn't a scientific formula, it's a behavior. Your own personality and individual preferences play an enormous role in what and how much you choose to eat. So before you can develop your own eating plan, you have to understand your own behaviors. Look at the food personalities and see which one(s) are familiar to you. Are you an emotional eater? A volume eater? A fruit juice lover? A snack lover? You can't change a behavior unless you first acknowledge it and learn to work with it. An honest assessment will also help you develop a food program that you can live with for the long haul. There's absolutely no reason to go on an eating plan you don't like; it will only lead to frustration and, eventually, failure. Your own food plan will help you avoid overeating and a sense of deprivation. You probably know that there is no generic food plan that works for everyone; if there was, we certainly would have found it by now. In this case, there is no one-size-fits-all plan.

common portion personalities

Here are some common Portion Personalities. See which one or ones best describe you, and use the solutions to tailor your eating plan.

VOLUME EATER

If you want quantity over quality, or more of the foods you feel neutral about rather than less of the foods you love, you are a Volume Eater. You want your food to look like a lot, to have some heft so that you feel full and satisfied.

Volume Scenario 1: Give me a heaping plate every time. It sure beats looking at a plate with a few tiny slices of meat in the center and then a lot of empty space.

Solution: If you enjoy a full plate, pile on the veggies—a heaping mound of veggies is okay any day, and you don't have to worry so much about portion sizes when you eat veggies, which are so nutrient-dense. Try to fill up at least half of your plate with veggies. The rest can be protein, such as chicken and fish, and starch. You also can pile on fruits and salads (without a lot of fatty salad dressings).

Volume Scenario 2: I need a lot to make me feel full. I can't eat dainty portions of anything. I want more, more, more, especially when it comes to snacks—I can easily eat a whole big bag of chips or pretzels.

Solution: Popcorn is a great volume snack. You can have 3 cups (3 baseballs) of unbuttered popcorn. That equals only 1 grain serving, so you still can have several other grains throughout the day. Another solution is to eat a single-serving (1-ounce) bag of chips or pretzels and avoid bringing jumbo bags into the house. You also can add fresh fruits and veggies as a snack to add volume.

Volume Scenario 3: I need a big breakfast, and I've heard that it's bad to start your day with starch. I like a lot of cereal. What do you recommend?

Solution: There is nothing wrong with including some starch at breakfast. The key is to include a healthy starch, such as whole-grain cereal, and try to include some protein as well, such as fat-free milk, yogurt, or eggs. When it comes to cereal, puff it up. Pile on puffed wheat or puffed brown rice cereal. You can have 2 cups (2 baseballs) of puffed wheat, which adds up to only 1 grain serving. Skip calorically dense cereals like granola—1 grain serving of granola is only ¼ cup (1 golf ball)!—and you will be fine. And it's okay to have a serving of fruit at breakfast—½ cantaloupe, a peach, or a banana. Fruit adds bulk and color, not to mention nutrients.

Volume Scenario 4: Desserts always stymie me on a diet. I want a big dessert, and almost every diet, especially the new low-carb ones, prohibits most desserts. What should I do?

Solution: It's fine to have a soft-serve frozen yogurt for dessert, especially if it satisfies you and helps you from grazing for something that feeds your cravings. Just be mindful of other treats and sugars during the day, and avoid large portions of whole-milk desserts, like ice cream. If ½ cup (½ baseball) of ice cream looks like nothing to you, skip it and opt for the frozen yogurt. But if you enjoy the taste of ice cream and can stop after one serving, have ½ cup (½ baseball) and add berries and fruits to make the dessert look bigger. The same goes for a sliver of cake or a chocolate chip cookie. Have a small sweet treat, and surround it with assorted fruits such as berries, melon, or grapes to make it seem like it's more.

Cheat Sheet for Volume Eaters

• All nonstarchy veggies are free. You can fill up on them. Steamed or microwaved is best. If you want them sautéed in oil, be sure to have half a walnut (1 tablespoon), that's it. Just because you can eat unlimited amounts of salad and vegetables doesn't mean you should use unlimited dressings and sauces.

• Eat carrots and beets instead of drinking carrot or beet juice. V8 and tomato juice, however, are very low in calories. It's okay if you're not meticulous about your portion.

• Fill up on low-cal fruits such as strawberries, blueberries, and melons such as cantaloupe. You can't have unlimited fruits, but if you want to have an extra portion, do it with fruits you can chew, not fruit juices.

• Note the bigger serving sizes for puffy starches: popcorn, puffed wheat, and puffed rice cereal, rice cakes. See Chapter 7 for more ways to pump up the volume.

- Choose smart volume snacks: soft-serve frozen yogurt, flavored rice cakes, soy crisps.
- Fill up on broth and tomato-based vegetable soups.
- You're better off with corn on the cob, a baked sweet potato, or a baked potato than with pasta—you only have one, and then you are done.
- Try sugar-free Jell-O or frozen fruit pops. They're mostly water.

LOPSIDED EATER

Did you get to the end of your Portion Teller Diary for the week and find out that you are heavy on one food group—be it grains, meat, fat, and so on—and light on all the rest? Then you're a Lopsided Eater, and you need to balance your food groups.

Lopsided Scenario 1: I just love a good steak. I can eat one for lunch and another at dinner, and still not be sick of it. It's the most perfect food in the world. And when I'm not having steak, I at least want a nice piece of meat.

Lopsided Scenario 2: I can't imagine a meal without bread—a bagel for breakfast, a sandwich for lunch, a pretzel or some other crunchy snack in the afternoon, and pasta and a few slices of garlic bread at dinner, not to mention the cookie for dessert.

Lopsided Scenario 3: Give me anything creamy and rich—I love French salad dressing, creamy soups, butter on my bread, sauces on fish and meat, and, of course, anything creamy and yummy for dessert, especially chocolate mousse with whipped cream.

The Solution to All Three Scenarios: Truth be told, other than steamed veggies and plain salad, you just can't eat huge amounts of any food group and lose weight. The solution to being a lopsided eater is first to become aware of your lopsided situation and which food group you're overeating. Next you need to choose how you would like to spread out your servings during the day.

In Scenario 1 (the meat overload), you can choose to have a nice-size steak for dinner if you opt for nonmeat sources of protein, such as meat alternatives or low-fat dairy, early in the day—beans, bean soup, eggs, low-fat yogurt, and cheese.

In Scenario 2 (the grain overload), if you want breads at each meal, try to skip bagels or muffins in the morning. Eating either would account for most of your grains for the day all in one meal. You may be better off choosing whole-grain cereal, bread, and brown rice during the course of the day and even allowing for an occasional handful of pretzels. And skip the garlic bread if you're opting for a pasta entrée.

In Scenario 3 (the fat overload), remember that fat is fattening, so pick and choose which fat you want most and work it into your plan. A little bit goes a long way in terms of adding flavor and zest to your meal.

Another problem with lopsided eating, or overeating from one food group, is that often it means that you are undereating from another food group. After you've kept your food diary for a while, you will spot which groups you are skimping on and can add foods from that group to your eating plan. Often people who overeat meat skimp on dairy. Those who overeat starch often skimp on fruit. My client Lindsay ate too many starches because she said she was hungry, but once she pumped up the fruits, she wasn't hungry anymore.

CAN'T-LIVE-WITHOUT EATER

Are there a few foods that you can't—or don't want to—live without? Is it absolutely essential to have a muffin for breakfast, or a special kind of yogurt, or a juicy hamburger on a kaiser roll? Are these foods that have been forbidden on other diets, which robbed you of the joy of your special beloved food? If so, you're a Can't-Live-Without Eater, and you need to learn to incorporate your must-haves into a healthful diet.

Can't-Live-Without Scenario 1: I can't live without cream-top maple-flavored yogurt. I know it's fatty (there's an entire layer of cream on the top) and has lots of added sugar, but it's one of the few foods I love. It feeds my soul and satisfies me. I would rather have a few bites of that, three times a week, than a lot of low-fat or nonfat yogurt, which doesn't do it for me.

Solution: Once a week replace low-fat yogurt, peanut butter, and fruit jam with cream-top maple yogurt. And because the fat in the yogurt is whole milk, or unhealthy fat, be conscious of red meat, butter, and other high-fat foods during the day.

Can't-Live-Without Scenario 2: I love croissants. But more than that, I love croissants that have sweet and sticky almonds on them. I know they are a sugar and grain fest and have almost no nutritional value, but I can't imagine not eating them every once in a while. Every other diet I've been on tells me I can't ever have them again.

Solution: Almond croissants are okay to have on occasion—honestly, how many breakfasts of whole-wheat toast and Cheerios can you have? Just smart-size it! Set aside one "free day" to have this treat. Make sure to watch both your grain and fat intake during the day. Also, note that the croissant has no fiber, so be sure to include fruit and veggies during the day, and have a small portion of a healthful grain in the evening, such as sweet potato or brown rice.

CHEATER

No matter how good my intentions are, I never eat according to plan. I eat more, or badly. I've cheated on every diet I've ever tried.

Cheater Solution: Remember, *The Portion Teller* isn't a diet. It's a new way of looking at your food. Examine the Portion Personalities to identify your specific habits. In general, if you overeat, don't react by starving yourself. If you cheat, return to the plan, reduce portions for the next two days, and exercise a bit more. If you feel deprived, you'll just overeat again.

• reality check— forbidden food •

Instead of putting your favorite food on the forbidden list, legalize it. That is, select your favorite food and make an allowance for it in your eating plan. Once it's a "legal" food, you don't have to feel deprived anymore or feel like you're "cheating," which often brings on a binge. Once it's legal, it's just another food on your food plan.

THE BAGEL LOVER

I know that a bagel is 5 grain servings, but I want it all the same.

Solution: Have the bagel, and go easy on the grains for the rest of the day. Or smartsize it! Scoop out the inside of the bagel—the doughy part—which is equivalent to 3 grains. That still leaves a couple more grain servings to include with dinner, such as some brown rice or kasha.

THE FRUIT JUICE LOVER

I've been told that fruit juice is high in sugar, but I like to have it in the morning.

Solution: That's okay, on occasion, as long as you account for it. As you will see in the next chapter, in sample breakfasts 1 and 2, skip the whole fruit and have the juice. The key is to have a 6-ounce glass (about the size of a 6-ounce yogurt container). And since juice doesn't provide much fiber, be sure to include some extra veggies and some fruit during the rest of the day. Just remember that fruit juice does contain sugar and calories. A little bit goes a long way.

THE SIDE DISHES LOVER

Give me a potato or some rice with dinner. A piece of meat or fish alone doesn't satisfy me; I need to have a side, especially something starchy. Veggies alone don't do the trick for me.

Solution: Skip the bread basket. Watch breads and cereals earlier in the day. You may find that you can do without starch for breakfast or lunch. You may be satisfied with an egg-white omelet or a yogurt and fresh fruit for breakfast instead of a bowl of cereal. And for lunch, you may prefer a salad instead of a sandwich.

THE PASTA LOVER

I have to have my pasta. I really enjoy Italian restaurants, and what's Italian without pasta?

Solution: Plan ahead by staying away from the sandwich and bread in sample lunches 1 and 2 as you will see in the next chapter. At lunch, concentrate on protein and veggies, such as grilled chicken, salmon, turkey, or beans over greens and veggies. At dinner, avoid the bread basket and starchy vegetables. Or, if you don't want to give up the grains during the day, when dining at your favorite Italian restaurant, order an appetizer-size portion or split an entrée size with a friend. And still stay away from the bread basket and the garlic bread.

the time factor

What is your favorite meal of the day, and why? Are there certain foods you feel you have to have at certain times of the day? A latte in the morning, or a glass of milk at night? Some granola at breakfast or in the afternoon? A glass of wine with dinner? A sandwich at lunch? A plate of pasta at dinner? An after-dinner sweet treat? Although it's better to eat more earlier in the day than later, you may prefer a larger dinner (rather than lunch) or an after-dinner snack. Think about what makes you feel satisfied, and when. The next few Portion Personalities are time-sensitive.

WHEN-TO-HAVE-MY-GRAINS QUANDARY

When do you want to eat your grains? A little at each meal, or would you rather have a larger amount for one or two of your meals? Would you prefer a sandwich at lunch or a pasta entrée, or do you want to have some crunchy snacks during the day? My client Larry can't make it through the day without those fat, Bavarian pretzels at about four in the afternoon.

Solution 1: Larry skips grains at breakfast and lunch so that he can have a handful of pretzels as a snack, and he enjoys a bowl of rice as a side dish at dinner. At breakfast, he prefers an egg-white omelet with fresh fruit to cereal. And for lunch, he likes a turkey burger without the bun and a side of grilled vegetables.

Solution 2: Murray can't live without his morning muffin, so he uses up most of his grains in the morning. He prefers a custom-blend salad with protein instead of a sandwich at lunch anyway. As a snack, he loves fruit salad, which he picks up at his favorite deli. At dinner, he skips the bread and potatoes.

Solution 3: Caroline, a sixteen-year-old who has lost and kept off over thirty pounds, loves a pasta entrée. She smartsizes it by saving up her grains during the day so that she can eat more than ½ cup (½ baseball) of pasta when dining out. She has 1 cup (1 baseball) of cereal in the morning, a salad with turkey at lunch, fresh fruit and peanut butter or a frozen yogurt with berries for her snack. She forgoes pretzels and crackers, which she can live without.

BREAKFAST HATER

People say "Breakfast is the most important meal" and "Never skip breakfast." But I don't want to eat first thing in the morning. I'm not hungry, and I'm always in a rush to get out of the house.

Solution: No problem. You don't have to eat a hearty breakfast first thing in the morning. It's okay to have it a little later, say midmorning. Just be sure not to skip it altogether. One option is to bring food to work so that you won't be tempted by the doughnuts or breakfast buns at your local coffee cart. Bring a low-fat yogurt or a hard-boiled egg with a piece of fruit, or half an English muffin with a little peanut butter. Try to include some protein (milk, yogurt, or cheese, a hard-boiled egg, etc.) to curb hunger. And make an effort not to go hours without eating. It is also worth exploring why you are not hungry in the morning. One possibility is that you overeat late at night. Be mindful of the late-night munching and try to train yourself to stop at one evening snack.

Take note if you have children, though: It's not a good idea to let them leave the house without breakfast because they usually don't have the option of eating midmorning—they have to wait until lunch.

DINNER LOVER

My most important meal is dinner. I've never liked lunch too much, but I love to eat a hearty dinner. But I've heard that you shouldn't load up at night.

Solution: You shouldn't "load up" for any meal, but if you prefer a smaller lunch and a larger dinner, that is okay. You will not gain weight if you watch your portions. But be sure not to skip meals during the day.

• portion patrol•

Help! I've heard that you should eat dinner by 6 P.M. I often work late. Should I skip dinner altogether?

You won't gain weight if you practice portion control throughout the day. It is best not to eat a large dinner late at night or one to two hours before going to sleep. If you know you have to eat a late dinner, have a snack in the late afternoon. Then have a light dinner, such as grilled fish and vegetables, or chicken or turkey breast over greens, soup, and salad, or a veggie burger in a small whole-wheat pita. Stick with fresh fruit, such as mixed berries or melon salads, as an after-dinner snack.

SNACK LOVER

I have got to have my afternoon and/or late-night snacks.

Solution: If you enjoy snacking, save up a fruit and maybe a dairy to have as a snack. Also, save your treats and sweets for a snack. Have a treat an hour or two after dinner so that you can look forward to it—unless, of course, you go to a restaurant that has your most favorite dessert.

SPECIAL-OCCASION VICTIM

My job requires me to go to a lot of events—buffets, cocktail parties, travel— and I can't stay away from salty nuts, hunks of cheese, and so on.

Solution: Eat a little something before you go to an event so that you're not starving: A salad, soup, some fruit, or yogurt is a great choice. You also can plan ahead so that you factor in a "treat" at the party. For example, you can have a few wedges of cheese as long as you are mindful of fats and dairy dur-ing the day. A handful of nuts is also okay. Pay attention to amounts. Take 1 Portion Teller serving and stop there.

"SEE-FOOD" EATER

Every time I go somewhere where everyone is eating—the ball park, a movie theater, an amusement park—I can't stop myself. I have to get a big bag of popcorn, some hot dogs, a soft-serve ice cream, whatever everyone else is eat-ing. I see it, and I have to have it.

Solution: Eat the smallest amount of popcorn you can order. Share the small size if possible. Eat a snack before you go to your favorite "see-food" event, so that you're not famished when you arrive. Or plan for it, and save up for the treat. Before you order it, ask yourself: Am I really hungry?

ALL-DAY NIBBLER/MINDLESS MUNCHER

I'm a stay-at-home mother and take a bite of everything—the kids' lunches as I'm making them, a spoonful of sauce for the pasta, a taste here and a taste there, and I'm gaining weight.

Solution: Plan your meals in advance. Do not eat when standing up. Don't pick at your children's food. Taste while cooking only *once* for seasoning and doneness. Have a healthy snack before your husband comes home, perhaps when the kids are eating, so that you're not overly hungry when you both sit down to eat. Have plenty of healthy snacks on hand. And perhaps the most important tip: Eat a satisfying portion. Don't deprive yourself with tiny portions that will only lead to picking and overeating throughout the day. Lots of little slivers add up to a huge slab. Be mindful.

TRIGGER VICTIMS

Trigger Scenario 1: If I have a sliver of cake, I'll go crazy and want more. I just can't stop at a small piece.

Solution: Don't have cake. If it's a tease, you know you have to steer clear of it. Instead, have something you like that is sweet but healthier—some caramel rice cakes, one or two graham crackers with a schmear of peanut butter and jam, a sweet fruit such as watermelon or grapes, or a serving of dried

• reality check—self-deception •

Here are some common situations when we eat more than we think.

- *I'll just have a sliver of cake.* You cut a tiny sliver, and eat, cut, and eat, and before you know it, you've eaten half the cake.

- *I'll only eat the broken pieces or the crumbs that fall off.* You know they add up!

- *I'll just have one.* And then you pick the biggest muffin you can find.

- *I'm not very hungry, so I'll just have a spoonful in front of the fridge.* And all of a sudden, the whole carton is gone.

- *I'm not going to order dessert.* You tell your dinner companion to get one dessert and two forks. But you end up having more than your friend. Beware: Those forkfuls count.

- *I'll just grab a few chips from the bag and put it back.* But a few handfuls later, you see that you had half a big bag, which is easy to forget when you close the bag and put it away. After all, you tell yourself, there's still half a bag left.

fruit. Another Portion Teller option is taking a sliver of cake with a generous side helping of fresh fruit; it makes the whole portion look a lot bigger. Or you can have one cookie so that you eat one unit only—you won't keep cutting a little sliver here, a little sliver there, until you've eaten more than half a cake. You also can freeze fruit, which turns it into a delicious ice-creamy snack. Spread some peanut butter on a banana, add some granola, and freeze. Frozen grapes are also a nice icy treat.

Trigger Scenario 2: I can't possibly eat cereal—if I have one bowl, I'll have a dozen. Stopping at one cup is unthinkable. Once I pour, I just keep pouring.

Solution: Stay away from cold cereal. Opt for an egg-white omelet on a slice of whole-wheat toast. Another option is oatmeal, which you're much less likely to overeat. Or try purchasing single-serving 1-ounce boxes of cereal.

BINGE EATERS

No matter whether it's chips, ice cream, or cereal, I end up eating it all, even if it's a big bag or box.

Solution: The best way to avoid bingeing is to not get started. If you don't have that first bite, you can't get going. One way is to keep your binge foods out of the house. If you would like to keep them around because other family members like them, buy single-serve products, such as individual boxes of cereal or single-serve bags of pretzels. Open one, and one only, and put the rest away. Instead of buying a half-gallon of ice cream, buy single-serve fudge pops or ice cream sandwiches. When you have to open a wrapper, you gain the psychological satisfaction of having eaten. Also, there's something about seeing the empty wrapper that reminds you that you've eaten it.

EMOTIONAL EATER

I turn to foods like brownies or macaroni and cheese for comfort. I have crav‑
ings at certain times in my menstrual cycle. I often eat when I am sad or
lonely.

Solution: If you know that you're an emotional eater, try to figure out a
nonfood response to your emotions. Shop, go to a movie, call a friend, exer‑
cise. Stop and think before you binge. You can allow yourself a treat, but take
the time to decide how much is reasonable and stop there.

STRESS EATERS

If I have a big meeting at work the next day, I stuff myself the night before
and wake up in a food stupor. Or if the kids are driving me crazy, I know I
need a big bowl of comfort food, such as ice cream. It calms me down.

Solution: The first thing to do is recognize when you're eating out of stress.
In the next chapter, I suggest keeping a Hunger Meter on your Portion Teller
Diary so you can see if you're eating without being hungry. If this is the case,
try to pile on veggies and fruit—foods that have a lot of volume and some
crunch to them, which may satisfy you. If you have to eat something out of
stress, make sure you have to think about it and travel to get it instead of just
opening the cupboard. By the time you put your coat on and walk out the
door, you may have taken a few deep breaths and lost the urge. But if you do
overeat one day, remember to cut back a little the next day and that all is not
lost. It's just another day. Avoid the all-or-nothing mentality.

BOREDOM EATERS

I can't watch TV without snacking. I'm not even hungry, but it's like being at a movie all night, every night—I need my nibble.

Solution: Plan ahead! Save up your grain servings for your snacks and have 3 or 4 cups of popcorn, a couple handfuls of pretzels, or a cup of frozen yogurt or sorbet. If you know you want to eat at night in front of the TV, make sure you don't finish your servings earlier in the day—save 1 fruit, 2 grains, or 1 dairy for TV time.

• reality check—tv •

If you can't sit in front of the TV without constant munching on snacks and loading up on drinks, declare a "No-Food Zone" on particular nights. If, say, Thursday is the night of your favorite TV lineup, it may be must-see TV night, but it's not snacking night—it's the No-Food Zone! Remind yourself: You'll miss out on must-see TV if you're too busy eating.

becoming a portion teller

Now that you have given some thought to your eating patterns and you've seen solutions for common pitfalls, take a moment to see where you are with estimating portions. This is a very important part of smartsizing. Where are you in managing your portions and understanding how they work in real life for you? Have you thought about portion size and what differentiates it from a serving size? Do you know that a deck of cards is approximately 3 ounces, which is 1 standard serving, or is this still something you have to think about?

If this is all new, work on educating yourself. Decide if measuring your food at home is a good exercise for you to do, even once, so that you can train yourself to "eyeball" portion sizes. Are you the type who would never measure anything—it's just not in your nature? Are you more visual? Then focus on the visuals from Chapter 2 and Appendix D, and take the time to pull together the objects discussed, line them up, and understand how they look in three dimensions so you can easily compare them to your portions. The following objects would be helpful: deck of cards, baseball, tennis ball, golf ball, shot glass, walnut, postal stamp, cap on a water bottle, 4 dice, CD and CD case, and a computer mouse. Or you may decide that sticking to the Portion Teller Diary is the way to go when it comes to managing your portions—you can break your eating habits into servings per food group and simply add them up at the end of the day to keep track. Maybe you'll find that neither measuring nor counting is your thing and that you'd prefer to work on visually guesstimating portion size and simply eating less.

Once you have a certain degree of portion-size awareness, ask yourself whether you are putting your knowledge into action. Perhaps you thought that a portion the size of a deck of cards (3 ounces) was all you were supposed to eat and said, "Forget it, I can't go on that diet." Or maybe you read that a bagel is 5 grain servings, and you thought you had to cut out all bagels, or even all grains, forever. Remember, this is not the case. There is no such thing as one portion size that is right for everybody. It's okay for you to pick and choose your portion, just as long as you understand how much food you can have from each food group throughout the day. You can include the occasional bagel, and you don't have to have a puny 3-ounce steak. It's awareness that matters.

• get smart! •

Which person best describes your ability to estimate your portions?

Person 1: I have no problem measuring out my portions the first few times to get used to portion sizes and relying on the visuals. I want to put this Portion Teller awareness into practice as much as possible. I have already put aside a golf ball, a baseball, a CD, and a deck of cards.

Person 2: I will never measure anything. It's too time-consuming, and I never eat at home anyway. I can see trying to put the visuals into practice, but I'm not very good at that kind of thing. My solution? I'm going to focus on eating a little bit less at each meal, by sharing my entrée in a restaurant, leaving a few bites on my plate, and taking a few turkey slices off my sandwich. I'm going to trim off what I can do without.

Person 3: There's no way I'm going to eat smaller portions—it just won't happen. I've decided to target my problem food—grains—and eat them less often. I'm going to eat grains at only two of my three meals and never as a snack, so that I don't have to worry so much about smartsizing portions all the time.

the portion teller eating plan

Never eat more than you can lift.

• MISS PIGGY

a baseline plan

nce you've been keeping the Portion Teller Diary for a week and you've evaluated your Portion Personality, it's time to start tailoring your diet according to what you've found. Before we build your personalized eating plan, let's start with a no-frills eating plan that provides a framework or structure that we can build on. This is nothing fancy—just a simple, straightforward meal plan that almost anyone would lose weight on. But only if they could stand it. And let's be realistic—it's just too dull to live a cottage cheese and celery existence. We're people, not machines, and few of us look at food as merely fuel. The baseline plan doesn't take into account your likes and dislikes, and would be repetitive and too structured to follow over the long haul. Eating should be a pleasure, not a chore.

But before we add the personal bells and whistles, we need to start with the basics. You may see several sample meals on this list that you like, as well as those that don't appeal to you. Choose the meals that are both practical and satisfying to you, and then you can start to make substitutions that work for you. Think of this plan as a mannequin, a basic form; once it's in place, you can begin to dress it up and personalize it with your own style. See Appendix E for additional Portion Teller Meal Plans.

sample meals

SAMPLE BREAKFAST 1:
Bran flakes with milk and mixed berries

SIZING UP YOUR SERVINGS

	VISUALS	HANDY METHOD
BRAN FLAKES	1 baseball	1 fist
MILK	8-ounce yogurt container	2 cupped hands
MIXED BERRIES	1 baseball	1 fist
WHEAT GERM (OPTIONAL)	½ walnut	3 thumb tips

1 cup bran flakes

1 cup skim milk or 1% milk or vanilla-flavored soy milk

1 cup mixed berries (blueberries, raspberries) or 3 tablespoons raisins

1 tablespoon wheat germ, optional

1 teaspoon brown sugar, optional

SAMPLE BREAKFAST 2:
Whole-grain toast or waffle with peanut butter and jam, and a banana

SIZING UP YOUR SERVINGS

	VISUALS	HANDY METHOD
SLICE TOAST OR WAFFLE	CD case or diameter of a CD	
PEANUT BUTTER	1/2 walnut	3 thumb tips
JAM	1-2 standard postal stamps	1-2 thumb tips

1 slice whole-grain toast or 1 whole-grain waffle

1 tablespoon peanut butter

1-2 teaspoons all-fruit jam, optional

1 banana

SAMPLE LUNCH 1:

Tossed salad platter with choice of protein (tuna, beans, or cheese)

SIZING UP YOUR SERVINGS

	VISUALS	HANDY METHOD
SALAD	2 baseballs	2 fists
SALAD DRESSING	½ shot glass	3 thumb tips
PROTEIN CHOICE (SELECT 1):		
TUNA (CANNED OR GRILLED)	1 deck of cards	your palm
LENTILS OR CHICK PEAS	1 baseball	1 fist
2 SLICES CHEESE	8 dice	2 fingers
1 SLICE WHOLE-GRAIN BREAD	CD case	

Tossed salad platter:

Mixed salad with your favorite vegetables (2 cups)

Choice of protein: 3 ounces canned tuna packed in water (small can) or fresh grilled tuna OR 1 cup lentils/beans of choice OR 2 slices part-skim cheese (2 ounces)

1 tablespoon Italian salad dressing OR olive oil, balsamic vinegar, and fresh lemon

1 slice whole-grain bread OR 2–3 whole-grain crisp breads (Ryvita, Kavli), optional

SAMPLE LUNCH 2:
Turkey sandwich on rye bread

SIZING UP YOUR SERVINGS

	VISUALS	HANDY METHOD
TURKEY BREAST	1 deck of cards	your palm
2 SLICES RYE BREAD	2 CD cases	
MAYONNAISE	½ walnut	3 thumb tips
LETTUCE AND TOMATO	½ baseball	handful

3 ounces turkey breast on 2 slices rye bread with 1 tablespoon mayonnaise topped with lettuce and tomato

Mustard, as desired

SAMPLE SNACK 1:
Yogurt with granola and an apple

SIZING UP SERVINGS

	VISUALS	HANDY METHOD
YOGURT	1 yogurt container	2 cupped hands
GRANOLA	1 golf ball	1 layer of your hand
APPLE	1 baseball	1 fist

6–8 ounces yogurt with ¼ cup granola and an apple

SAMPLE SNACK 2:

Popcorn and string cheese

SIZING UP YOUR SERVINGS

	VISUALS	HANDY METHOD
3 CUPS AIR-POPPED POPCORN	3 baseballs	3 fists
1 STRING CHEESE (1 OZ)	4 dice	1 finger

3 cups air-popped popcorn and 1 ounce string cheese

SAMPLE DINNER 1:

Chopped salad to start; broiled flounder with mixed vegetables and whole-wheat pasta topped with fresh tomato sauce

SIZING UP YOUR SERVINGS

	VISUALS	HANDY METHOD
TOSSED SALAD	2 baseballs	2 fists
OLIVE OIL	1/2 shot glass	3 thumb tips
BROILED FLOUNDER	1 checkbook	length of hand including palm and fingers
MIXED VEGGIES	1 baseball	1 fist or 2 cupped hands
DRIZZLE OLIVE OIL	1 water bottle cap	1 thumb tip
PASTA	1 baseball	1 fist or 2 cupped hands
TOMATO SAUCE	1/2 baseball	1 handful
PARMESAN CHEESE	1/2 walnut	3 thumb tips

2 cups chopped salad with 1 tablespoon olive oil and balsamic vinegar (as much as you want), and spices

3–4 ounces flounder or filet of sole broiled or baked with lemon, parsley, spices, and 1 teaspoon oil or butter

Steamed vegetables seasoned with drizzle (1–2 teaspoons) olive oil and fresh garlic

1 cup cooked whole-wheat pasta topped with ½ cup fresh tomato sauce and 1 tablespoon fresh Parmesan cheese

SAMPLE DINNER 2:

Vegetable soup to start; chicken stir-fry with mixed vegetables and brown rice

SIZING UP YOUR SERVINGS

	VISUALS	HANDY METHOD
VEGETABLE SOUP	1 baseball	1 fist or 2 cupped hands
CHICKEN BREAST	2 decks of cards	2 palms
VEGGIES	1 baseball	1 fist
OIL	½ shot glass	3 thumb tips
BROWN RICE	1 baseball	1 fist

1 cup vegetable soup

Chicken stir-fry:

6-ounce grilled or broiled chicken breast

1 cup stir-fried vegetables (mixed veggies with 1 tablespoon sesame or peanut oil)

1 cup brown rice

SAMPLE SNACK 1:

Frozen yogurt topped with nuts or raisins

SIZING UP YOUR SERVINGS

	VISUALS	HANDY METHOD
FROZEN YOGURT	1 baseball	1 fist
MIXED NUTS	1 golf ball	1 layer of your hand
RAISINS	1 golf ball	1 layer of your hand

1 cup frozen yogurt topped with 1 ounce nuts OR 3–4 tablespoons raisins

SAMPLE SNACK 2:

Fruit salad and a rice cake with a schmear of peanut butter

SIZING UP YOUR SERVINGS

	VISUALS	HANDY METHOD
FRUIT SALAD	1 baseball	2 handfuls
PEANUT BUTTER	$\frac{1}{2}$ walnut	3 thumb tips
RICE CAKE	CD diameter	1 palm

1 cup fruit salad and 1 rice cake with 1 tablespoon peanut butter

the portion teller diary

Now that you have the basics, it's time to make some changes. Using the sample menus as a starting point, start adjusting your food plan using what you've learned. Track your progress in the Portion Teller Diary.

ten simple steps

Remember the eight simple steps to keeping the Portion Teller Diary (see page 100)? Now there are two new ones.

1. Write down everything you eat.

2. Record your portion.

3. Place it in the right food group.

4. Break it into standard serving sizes.

5. Tally up the servings from each food group for the day.

6. Cross it off on the diary.

7. Don't forget to include water.

8. Write down what kind of exercise you do and for how long.

9. Record (and congratulate yourself) for your portion progress. If you are accustomed to having an entrée size of pasta at a restaurant and switched to an appetizer size, write it down! If you used to have a pint of orange juice for breakfast and switched to a fresh orange, record it! If you make the orange juice switch, you are saving almost 100 calories. If you make this change

daily, you will save 100 calories a day, which translates into a ten-pound loss over a year! Make a note of this change, so when you start losing weight, you'll know exactly why.

10. Assess your diet. Now that you've filled in the diary for the entire day, it's time to take stock of your eating program. Compare how much you ate from each food group to your Portion Target Numbers (see below to figure out your Portion Target Numbers). Ask yourself: Did I eat too many grains today and miss out on the fruits and veggies? Have I been indulging in more treats and sweets than I want? Is my diet too heavy on red meats and too light on fish and poultry? You can't make changes until you make an honest assessment of exactly where you are and where you want to be. Also take a look at the end of a week, and assess the entire week, and make a note of your progress and where you need to make changes. This is a learning process. Remember, you don't have to do it forever.

the portion teller diary

Remember, a blank Portion Teller Diary is in the back of the book. How long you decide to keep the diary is up to you. One month would be sufficient to increase your awareness and be able to assess your eating habits, since they may vary according to how much you dine out, your monthly moods and stresses, big events or occasions like cocktail and dinner parties, travel, and so on. If you think the month you've chosen to keep the Portion Teller Diary is representative, you can stop when it's over. If you want a more accurate snapshot of your eating habits over a period of months, keep the diary for a longer period of time.

your daily servings
for each food group

You probably noticed that I recommend a *range* of servings per day for each of the food groups: 3+ vegetables; 2 to 4 fruits; 4 to 8 grains and starchy vegetables; 2 to 3 dairy; 2 to 3 meats; 1 to 3 fats; and 0 to 2 treats and sweets. Now's the time to figure out the right number of servings that works for you, your Target Number. You will need to have these target numbers in mind when you fill out your Portion Teller Diary. The blank Portion Teller Diary that I've provided in the back of the book has the highest number of servings per day. Use the following factors to determine your target number of servings per day for each of the food groups. If your Target Number is lower, simply cross off the graphics in each food group *before you photocopy* the blank form so that you can see the correct number. For example, the grain group has 8 grain graphics. If your Portion Target Number for grains is 5, cross off 3 of the graphics before you copy the Portion Teller Diary and place it in your notebook. Do not go lower than the minimum number of servings per food group.

find your target numbers

To figure out your Target Numbers, consider these factors:

1. *Exercise level.* Exercise burns calories, so if you exercise regularly, you can eat a bit more. If you love to eat, you can buy yourself higher Target Numbers by increasing your exercise. If you are fairly sedentary, however, and spend all day sitting at work, your Target Numbers are at the low end. For example, the Portion Teller Pyramid recommends 2 to 4 servings of fruit per day. Two servings is the low end for fruit.

2. *Age.* If you are still growing, you can eat at the high end of the range. For example, the Portion Teller Pyramid recommends 2 to 3 servings of meats and meat alternatives per day. Three is the high end for meats and meat alternatives. Postmenopausal women may experience a drop in metabolism and suddenly find that they gain weight easily. If this is the case, choose Target Numbers at the low end of the scale.

3. *Gender.* Men generally can eat more than women and do not need to eat from the lower end of the recommended servings.

4. *Appetite.* If you are used to eating a lot, reducing your food intake drastically may be too much of a shock to your system. Start by making healthier food choices and gradually reduce the number of servings. And remember, it's OK to have plenty of nonstarchy vegetables.

5. *Amount of weight to lose.* If you need to lose only a few pounds, you should start with lower Target Numbers—fewer servings from each food group per day. If you have a lot of weight to lose, you can start with higher target numbers. Heavier people burn more calories per day—they use energy carrying around the extra weight. But if you know you have a sluggish metabolism, you may want to choose lower Target Numbers.

cheat chart for determining your target number

MINIMUM NO. OF SERVINGS PER FOOD GROUP	MIDDLE NO. OF SERVINGS PER FOOD GROUP	MAXIMUM NO. OF SERVINGS PER FOOD GROUP
Women over 50	Lower number makes you feel too hungry; you exercise at least 4 times per week	Growing teens
Sedentary women		Very active people
Smaller women with 5–10 pounds to lose		Men
		Larger people with over 50 pounds to lose

target number tips

Determining your Target Number is not a black-and-white issue. Adjust your plan up or down based on how you feel. If you aren't losing ½ to 1 pound per week, you can shift to the minimum number of servings. If you eat the minimum and are always hungry, increase the servings, or just increase vegetables and fruit. Play around to find what works. If you are following this plan correctly, you should not feel hungry.

Customize your numbers. If you love fruit and veggies, it's okay to add more of these food groups before you add more starch or meat. If you're feeling hungry, increase your Target Number for grains and starchy vegetables (and treats and sweets) last. Try eating more fruit and vegetables first. Same goes if you're a volume eater—eat more fruit and vegetables. If you love dairy but can do without starch, it's okay to have an extra dairy serving while keeping your starch to the minimum 4 servings. If you love breads, increase grains to 6 servings while keeping dairy and meat servings at 2. And if you know that having starch just makes you crave more starch or if you're bread phobic, then have the minimum of 4 grain/starchy vegetable servings and stick with whole grains and starchy vegetables such as butternut squash or baked potatoes.

And remember: The only food group you can leave out of your plan is treats and sweets!

• portion patrol•

Help! I overate on sweets today. How can I make up for it?

Get right back on track and don't starve yourself. Tomorrow make sure to have three structured meals and include protein, such as low-fat dairy, chicken, turkey, fish, or beans, at every meal. And be sure to include fiber-rich foods, such as fruits and vegetables. It's okay to go easy on the grains for a day or two. And skip the treats and sweets for a few days. But don't cut down on other food groups. And, if you are hungry, feel free to add a salad or steamed veggies.

Portion Teller Diary

FOOD (INCLUDE METHOD OF PREPARATION)	YOUR PORTION	FOOD GROUP	NUMBER OF SERVINGS
BREAKFAST:			
LUNCH:			
SNACK:			
DINNER:			
SNACK:			

FRUITS:

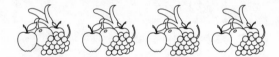

VEGETABLES:

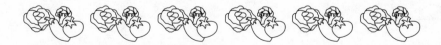

GRAINS AND STARCHY VEGETABLES:

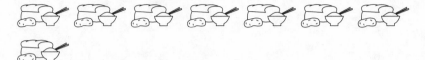

DAIRY:

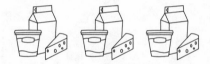

FISH, POULTRY, MEATS, AND MEAT ALTERNATIVES:

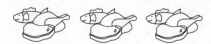

FATS:

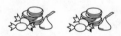

TREATS AND SWEETS:

WATER:

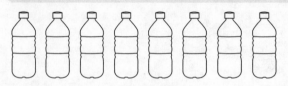

EXERCISE:

PORTION TELLER PROGRESS:

To help you understand how to fill out a Portion Teller Diary, here is a sample diary completed by my fictitious client Susie. Susie's diet is very simple and basic. I purposely did this to show how to record your portion, the food groups, and the standard serving sizes. Susie's diary is by no means a suggestion of what you should eat; it's just a sample we can look at together.

Susie's Portion Teller Diary

FOOD (INCLUDE METHOD OF PREPARATION)	YOUR PORTION	VISUAL	FOOD GROUP	NUMBER OF SERVINGS
BREAKFAST:				
Cheerios	1 cup	1 baseball	grain	1
Fat-free milk	1 cup	1 baseball	dairy	1
Blueberries and raspberries	1 cup	1 fist	fruit	1
LUNCH:				
Pita pocket sandwich:				
Whole-wheat pita	1-oz size	CD diameter	grain	1
Turkey breast	3 oz	palm	meat	1
Mixed veggies (shredded carrots, lettuce, tomato)	1 cup	1 baseball	vegetable	1
Honey mustard	1 Tbsp	$^1/_2$ walnut		
Vinaigrette dressing	1–2 tsp	1–2 thumb tips	fat	$^1/_2$
SNACK:				
Low-fat vanilla yogurt	8 ounces	1 container	dairy	1
Apple	1	1 tennis ball	fruit	1
Peanut butter	1 Tbsp	$^1/_2$ walnut	fat	1

DINNER:

Vegetable soup	12 oz	1 soda can	vegetable	$1^1/_2$
Grilled salmon	4–5 oz	$1\,^1/_2$ decks of cards	meat	$1^1/_2$
Baked sweet potato	1	1 computer mouse	grain/starchy vegetable	2
Grilled vegetables	1 cup	1 baseball	vegetable	2
Drizzle olive oil	1–2 tsps	1–2 thumb tips	fat	$^1/_2$

SNACK:

Fresh fruit salad	1 cup	2 cupped hands	fruit	1
Air-popped popcorn	3 cups	3 fists	grain	1
Chocolate Kisses	2 pieces		treats/sweets	$^1/_2$

Fruit 3	Dairy 2
Veggie $4^1/_2$	Fat 2
Grain 5	Treats/sweets $^1/_2$
Meat $2^1/_2$	

FRUITS:

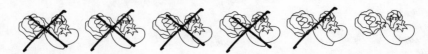

VEGETABLES:

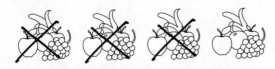

GRAINS AND STARCHY VEGETABLES:

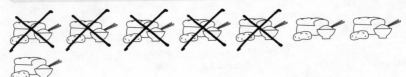

DAIRY:

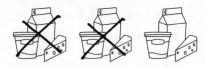

FISH, POULTRY, MEATS, AND MEAT ALTERNATIVES:

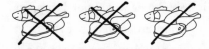

FATS:

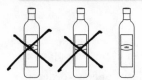

TREATS AND SWEETS:

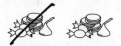

WATER:

Drank 4 glasses (32 oz) flavored seltzer and 4 glasses (32 oz) tap water.

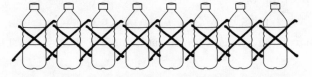

EXERCISE:

Walked briskly for 45 minutes. Lifted weights for 15 minutes.

PORTION TELLER PROGRESS:

Satisfied eating the regular-size pita (1 ounce) instead of the large pita (2 ounce) at lunch; saved 1 bread serving so I can have popcorn later.

Plan in advance. If you'll be eating dinner at a restaurant, eat a vegetarian pita for lunch (with 1 cup of your favorite bean salad instead of turkey in the pita), so that you can have a larger piece of fish in the restaurant.

how did susie fill out her diary? and how did susie do on her plan?

Breakfast: Susie poured about a baseball's worth of Cheerios into her bowl, which she knew from her visuals is about 1 cup, added 1 cup of milk, and then grabbed a fist's worth of berries, which she knew was about 1 cup, and dumped them in. Susie checked the serving chart and noted that she had 1 grain serving, 1 serving of dairy, 1 serving of fruit, and entered it into her diary. Before she ran to work, she grabbed a low-fat vanilla yogurt and an apple and put them in her tote bag.

Lunch: Susie went to her favorite take-out deli. Instead of picking up a premade sandwich which she knew would be jumbo-sized, she special-ordered a small whole-wheat pita with turkey breast, mixed veggies, and honey mustard, and asked for the vinaigrette salad dressing on the side. When she got back to her desk at work, she knew she had about a palm's worth, or about 3 ounces, of turkey, which is 1 serving of meat. The pita was the small size, the diameter of a CD, and, at about 1 ounce, equal to 1 grain serving. The veggies would fill out a baseball, so again, 1 cup, 1 serving. And she added her own salad dressing by splashing on about 1 to 2 teaspoons (about 1 to 2 thumb tips), which is ½ fat serving. She wrote it down on a note card so she could enter it into her diary when she got home that night.

Snack: Susie always, without fail, gets hungry around 4:00 P.M., and planned ahead for it. She kept her yogurt and apple in the office fridge. But she knows from experience that this low-cal snack wouldn't satisfy her craving for something a bit richer and more creamy. (In the past she used to have a peanut butter energy bar and a whole-milk yogurt.) So she put a glob of peanut butter (she keeps a jar in the office fridge) on her apple slices and enjoyed that small treat. She wrote down 1 dairy, 1 fruit, and 1 fat. (She used ½ a walnut's worth of peanut butter, or about 1 tablespoon, which is equal to 1 fat.) Susie continued recording the rest of her day in this manner.

Sizing Up Susie's Servings

How did Susie know how many servings she had? She sized them up with visuals from Appendix D. Here are a few examples:

1 cup Cheerios =   visual of 1 baseball

1 tablespoon peanut butter =   visual of ½ walnut

4-5 ounces grilled salmon =   visual of 1½ decks of cards

1 baked sweet potato =   visual of 1 computer mouse

3 cups popcorn =   visual of 3 fists

1 cup fresh fruit salad =   visual of 2 cupped hands

common portion traps

Susie did very well in terms of balancing the food groups on the first day she kept of her Portion Teller Diary. But how did she do in the next few days? Let us walk through a few of the most common portion traps. After you've kept your own diary for a few weeks, you will see that certain portion patterns emerge. The most common pattern is eating too much of your favorite foods, which often fall into one food group, rather than balancing your diet. You just may recognize some of your own eating pitfalls in Susie's daily diet blunders.

starch overload

On day 2 of keeping her food diary, Susie ate a bagel with cream cheese and a glass of orange juice for breakfast, take-out Chinese food for lunch (chicken and vegetables with white rice, but she skimped on her veggies), a hot pretzel from a street vendor as a snack on her way to a meeting, and a pasta entrée with two pieces of garlic bread at her favorite Italian restaurant for dinner. What is wrong with this picture?

Let's calculate her grain servings:

Bagel	5 ounces	5 grains
White Rice	2 cups	4 grains
Hot pretzel	6 ounces	6 grains
Pasta entrée	3 cups	6 grains
Garlic bread	2 slices	2 grains
Total number of grain servings = 23 servings.		

Whoa! Starch overload! Not only did Susie overdo the grains, she also picked white-flour products, meaning that she missed out on getting more healthy nutrients and fiber. She skimped on fresh fruits and vegetables, missing out on key nutrients such as vitamin C, folate, and potassium as well as phytonutrients and fiber. She also skipped dairy, missing out on calcium and protein.

HOW TO FIX THE STARCH OVERLOAD

Breakfast

- Skip the bagel and include some protein here. Have an egg-white omelet with fruit and 1 slice of whole-wheat toast for breakfast.
- If you absolutely want that bagel, watch your bread later in the day. And, to include some protein, choose melted part-skim mozzarella instead of the cream cheese.

Lunch

- Have only 1 cup of rice at lunch or skip it all together. Opt for brown rice to boost fiber. Be sure to eat all the vegetables.

Snack

- Have fresh fruit with yogurt as a midafternoon snack instead of the hot pretzel.

Dinner

- Skip the garlic bread and have a tossed salad, grilled veggies, or vegetable soup instead.
- Share the pasta.
- If you absolutely must have the pasta, work around it; watch bread earlier in the day.

protein overload

The following day Susie was sluggish. She blamed it on all that bread and decided to curb the grains and have more protein. She had a cheese omelet at a diner for breakfast. For lunch, she had an open-face turkey sandwich from a deli. For dinner, she ate out and had the 24-ounce porterhouse steak special, which came with a broccoli floret or two. What's wrong with this picture?

Let's calculate how many ounces of meat Susie had:

Cheese omelet	3 eggs (equivalent to 3 ounces)	1 meat
Turkey	6 ounces	2 meat
Steak	18 ounces (cooked)	6 meat

Total number of meat/poultry/fish (or alternatives) ounces consumed = 27 ounces. This is equivalent to 9 meat servings or three to four days' worth of meat.

Too much protein! By loading up on meats, Susie skimped on the fruits, veggies, dairy, and whole grains, which means a lack of fiber and nutrients.

HOW TO FIX THE PROTEIN OVERLOAD

Breakfast

- Eat an egg-white omelet or a hard-boiled egg at home. Or have a bowl of cereal and fruit or some yogurt and fresh fruit sprinkled with granola at the diner instead.

Lunch

- Share a turkey sandwich with a friend. Add a salad or a vegetable soup with your lunch.
- If you know you are eating at your favorite steakhouse for dinner, instead of the turkey sandwich, try for a meat alternative, such as a lentil soup or split pea soup, and a salad with whole-grain crackers, or a veggie burger in a whole-wheat pita with lettuce and tomato.

• portion patrol •

Help! I'm going to a steakhouse for dinner. How can I get my protein during the day?

It's okay to save your meat for dinner if you want to indulge in steak on occasion. You can get protein earlier in the day from low-fat dairy such as yogurt or cheese or milk, bean salads and bean soup, lentils, and eggs. When you go to the steakhouse, share a steak. Remember, you don't need to eat the whole cow!

Snack

- Have a fresh fruit for a snack.

Dinner

- Order the smallest steak you can find or share the porterhouse. Be sure to add a generous helping of veggies (not just a broccoli floret) and a mixed green salad. And remember, you do *not* have to finish the steak.

FAT FEST

Whatever Susie was doing over the past few days was not working. She was gaining weight instead of losing. Susie had heard her friends rave about high-fat, low-carb diets, so she decided to give it a try. Breakfast included 3 eggs cooked in butter with several strips of bacon. Lunch was a hamburger with melted cheese (no bun, of course). She snacked on handfuls of nuts, and dinner was a steak with French fries. What's wrong with this picture?

Let's see where the fat lies:

Butter in the eggs
Bacon
Burger
High-fat cheese
Nuts
Steak
French fries

This is a fat fest! This regimen is too low in carbs, especially the healthy carbs. It contains virtually no veggies, fruits, or whole grains, and thus is practically devoid of fiber as well as folate and potassium and antioxidants, such as vitamin C and beta carotene. This diet is also much too high in protein.

HOW TO FIX THE FAT FEST

Breakfast

- Prepare the eggs in olive oil spray instead of butter.
- Add fresh fruit with breakfast, such as an orange or one cup mixed berries.
- Skip the bacon.

Lunch

- Choose between the lunch burger and the dinner steak. And watch your portion size. Include turkey, chicken, or fish, tofu, or beans for the other meal. Salmon is a great choice of healthy omega-3 fatty acids; it certainly beats the saturated fat found in steak.
- Skip the melted high-fat cheese on the burger.

Snack

- Snack on fruit and yogurt, and enjoy a sprinkling of nuts as a topping, but watch the amount, especially on days where you already ate a lot of fat (a burger, high-fat cheese, etc.).

Dinner

- If you are having the steak, choose spinach sautéed in olive oil or a baked sweet potato instead of French fries. Start the meal with a tossed salad with colorful veggies or a vegetable soup.

custom-tailoring your portion teller program

After keeping Portion Teller Diaries for a while, people usually discover certain habits about themselves; patterns take shape and a distinct portion personality begins to emerge. Sometimes people find little quirks, small details that they never knew or thought about, like the unconscious desire to save their favorite bite of dinner until the last moment or the craving for something sweet before bed. Or it could be more significant, such as overeating protein or grains on a regular basis, or using eating out and occasions to splurge, to treat as a "special" day, even if they're eating out all the time. The Portion Teller Diary often leads to eating habit revelations, and it's these revelations that help you understand yourself so that you can build an eating plan that works for you.

You can eat what you like as long as you learn to pick and choose what

portion shockers . . .

- 78 percent of people surveyed by the American Institute for Cancer Research said that what they eat is more important than how much they eat for managing their weight.
- 69 percent of Americans belong to the clean-your-plate club.
- 42 percent of people base the amount they eat on what they are used to eating.
- Results from the Garbage Project, an analysis of household trash, revealed a huge discrepancy between what people say they eat and what they actually eat. They called it the "Lean Cuisine Syndrome": People tend to over-report foods that are good for them (such as fruits and veggies) but underreport foods that they consider bad for them.

and when you want to eat, to guesstimate how much you're actually eating, and to account for it. The key to smartsizing is understanding how much you can eat from each food group on a daily basis and breaking that amount down into an eating plan that is practical and satisfying. As long as your daily servings from each food group add up to your Target Numbers, you can maintain or lose weight without any feeling of deprivation.

• portion patrol •

Help! I love nuts, but I know they are fattening. Once I start eating them, I can't stop. Any suggestions?

If a food is a "trigger" for you and may lead you to overeat, it is best not to tempt fate. But nuts are healthy, so it's worth trying to train yourself to just have a little. Try purchasing nuts with the shells still on. Opening them takes time, so you'll end up eating more slowly and will feel full faster. The shells also will serve as a reminder of how many you've eaten, which will help you to avoid the mindless munching. If you can't get nuts with the shells still on, a great portion trick is to fill up an empty tin of Altoids with peanuts or almonds; a perfect one-ounce portion.

plan ahead!

No food is off limits as long as you know how to incorporate it into your food plan. If you plan ahead and adjust your thinking (and eating!) during the day, you can't go wrong. The key is to use your Portion Teller Diary to help you preplan your daily eating menu. If you know where you will be later in the day or tomorrow (or even a few days down the line), you can fill out your Portion Teller Diary in advance, taking into account your schedule. For example, if you know that you have to go to a work-related dinner at an Italian restaurant tomorrow night, you can plan ahead for a pasta entrée. Write it into your diary, and fill out the rest of the day accordingly: choose protein/fruit at breakfast and protein/veggies at lunch so that the pasta is part of the plan. Cross off each preplanned food as you eat it. Doing so is a very satisfying feeling.

think like a portion teller

The most important adjustment you can make is in your attitude. Abandon the old all-or-nothing syndrome that stops so many dieters from making progress. Celebrate small victories. Treat yourself when you make portion progress, but not with food—with smaller pants! And remember, take one day at a time. Developing portion-size awareness is a learning process. Focus on the small changes that you can live with for life.

portion teller diary fine-tuning

By now some of the changes to your eating plan should be starting to fall into place. You may be ready to do some fine-tuning. Let's look at a very common trouble spot: It's very easy to overeat with the temptations around us. So much of what, when, and why we eat has to do with what's around us—the aroma of food, the sight of it (as it is cooking or being served), the enticing advertisements and heaping portions—all these things can be very seductive and hard to resist. It's important not to let these outside influences get the better of you and your eating plan, undermining all of your progress. Here are a few tips for taking control of your environment and your own eating habits.

the hunger meter

How hungry are you when you eat? Do you have a tendency to eat out of boredom or stress, because "everyone else is," because you think you're supposed to? Whenever you smell something delicious? Do you often wait until you're famished and then eat everything in sight? Or do you stuff yourself so that you feel so full that you are about to burst? Do you know the difference between eating until you're satisfied or comfortable and eating until you're stuffed? Never allow yourself to become so famished that you're dizzy or so full that it hurts. Either extreme is unhealthy and both lead to out-of-control eating. You need to be able to recognize healthy hunger—that slight pang that tells you to eat—before you let yourself get so ravenous that you overeat. And you need to be able to recognize the difference between healthy fullness and being so stuffed that you're uncomfortable.

It's hard to gauge your hunger. Brian Wansink and colleagues from the University of Illinois provided people with a "bottomless" bowl of soup that filled slowly and continuously from a hole in the bowl, appearing never to empty. People didn't seem to notice—they just kept eating. In fact, they ate 40 percent more than the people who were fed normal-size bowls of soup. It's a challenge for people to recognize when they've had enough and to push their bowl or plate aside. People eat just because it's there or because they're served a bigger portion; so it's important to pay attention to our internal hunger mechanisms.

If eating without feeling hungry or constant eating is a real problem for you, you may find it helpful to use the Hunger Meter. Every time you eat something, rate your hunger on a scale of 1 to 5:

• portion patrol•

Help! I eat too quickly and then feel absolutely stuffed after a meal.

Train yourself to slow down by practicing these techniques:

- Cut your food into smaller pieces.

- Chew your food well.

- Put your fork and knife down between bites.

- If you're eating with others, enjoy the company.

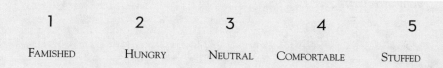

1	2	3	4	5
FAMISHED	HUNGRY	NEUTRAL	COMFORTABLE	STUFFED

Write the number next to what you ate in your Portion Teller Diary so that you can easily spot when you are eating for reasons other than hunger or when you are stuffing yourself. If you ate lunch when you weren't particularly hungry or full, give yourself a 3. If you went a little crazy at your nephew's graduation and ended up eating all afternoon long, write down what you ate and put a 5 next to your list of foods. Rating your hunger and fullness also will force you to think about whether you're hungry when you decide to grab a snack or nibble in front of the fridge. This is self-awareness in action!

graduate from the portion teller diary

Once you've kept the Portion Teller Diary long enough to get a grip on your eating habits, you may want to move away from the diary to the Portion Teller Progress Sheet. Instead of going "cold turkey" and giving up the diary for good, you can take this intermediate step: Rather than entering everything you eat into the diary, just calculate the number of servings from each food group you had during the course of the day and write the number on the progress sheet. To do this you need to know how your portion translates to standard serving sizes. Record this information however works best for you. You can carry around an index card for each day in your bag, enter it into your daily planner, keep a list on your computer, or use the kitchen chalk board or a wipe-off magnet board on the fridge. And remember, this is a learning process. It is okay to guesstimate. You don't have to be exact. The goal is to become more aware of what and approximately how much you are eating. Here is a sample of how to keep track with a Portion Teller Progress Sheet. Make copies of the Portion Teller Progress Sheet in Appendix C for your own use.

portion teller progress sheet

Record the number of servings per day consumed from each food group along with any portion progress for the week. Notice that the Portion Teller Progress Sheet begins on Monday.

FOOD GROUP	MON	TUES	WED	THURS	FRI	SAT	SUN
FRUITS: *2-4 servings daily*	3	4					
VEGETABLES: *3 + servings daily*	5	4					
GRAINS AND STARCHY VEGETABLES: *4-8 servings daily*	6	5					
DAIRY: *2-3 servings daily*	2	3					
FISH, POULTRY, MEATS, AND ALTERNATIVES: *2-3 servings daily*	2	2					
FATS: *1-3 servings daily*	2	1					
TREATS/SWEETS: *0-2 servings daily*	O	1					
PORTION TELLER PROGRESS:							

• get smart! •

CHOOSE WISELY

- Do eat as many nonstarchy veggies as you want.
- Order a salad or vegetable soup to start.
- Choose olive oil–based dressings rather than creamy varieties.
- Order dishes steamed, grilled, broiled, or baked.
- Order brown rice instead of white.
- Opt for grilled fish or chicken.
- At Italian restaurants, choose red sauce or marinara for pasta.
- Order primavera.
- Choose turkey and chicken as a sandwich filling over deli meats.
- Hold the mayo! Opt for mustard or ketchup instead.
- Choose whole-wheat or rye bread instead of white.
- Drink 6 to 8 glasses of water or seltzer daily.
- Order a baked potato, sweet potato, or brown rice instead of fries.
- Order fresh fruit, such as mixed berries, for dessert.
- Order coffee beverages with nonfat milk.
- Remember that fiber is filling.

KNOW YOUR LIMITS

- Limit cream sauces for pasta.
- Stay away from extra cheese.
- Limit red meat.
- Beware of fried dishes: fried chicken, egg rolls, tortilla chips, and so on.
- Remember that French fries count as a treat, not as a vegetable.
- Limit white bread products.
- Go easy on the sauces.
- Limit salad dressings, croutons, butter, and mayonnaise.
- Skip the soda.
- Eat cakes, pies, and cookies in moderation, even "low-carb" or "low-fat" ones.

smartsize your life

Stomachs shouldn't be waist baskets.

• P. J. THOMAJON

n o matter how much progress you make with your eating plan, there's no getting around the fact that we live in a culture that pushes more food on us at all times. This is a particular problem for "See-Food" Eaters, who eat because the food is there, not because they're hungry. But it's hard for everyone to resist the environmental and cultural signals to buy, order, and eat larger portions at every turn: the grocery store, restaurants, delis, sporting events, street fairs, dinner and cocktail parties, work events, buffets, and barbeques. In the United States, overeating is the norm rather than the exception. Now that you've developed portion-size awareness and know that you can't avoid the constant pressure to eat more, what are you supposed to do about it? This chapter gives you the tools to deal with portion pressure and provides tips, tricks, and activities to help you avoid portion pitfalls.

a smartsize way of life

I know I've said it before, but it's back to basics: Unless it is pure water, size matters. Bigger bites can cost you: A bigger portion, regardless of the food, contains more calories. Remember that an 8-ounce glass of soda contains 100 calories, while a 64-ounce Double Gulp contains close to 800 calories. Big portions cause weight gain. It's not an issue of too many carbs, fats, or protein. If eaten in excess, any of these nutrients will make you gain weight. No matter what eating plan you ultimately adopt, you still can lose weight painlessly by cutting back on your portions. Just smartsize it. One of my favorite food facts, one that I tell people over and over again, is that you can lose ten pounds a year by cutting back on 100 calories a day. That's a few less bites of a dessert, a handful less of potato chips, a couple of fork twirls less of pasta. To trim calories, just trim your portions. Remember, you want to make small lifestyle changes that you can live with. Instead of meticulously consulting calorie charts or obsessively checking the USDA Nutrient Database for Standard Reference, try these simple, painless, calorie-cutting moves.

SMARTSIZE WAYS TO ELIMINATE APPROXIMATELY 100 CALORIES

- Split a small order of French fries with a friend.
- Switch from a 20-ounce soda to a 12-ounce can.
- Eat only half of a candy bar or energy bar. (Sorry, energy bars have calories, even if the bars usually are touted as low-fat or low-carb health food.)
- Use 1 tablespoon of salad dressing instead of 2 tablespoons.
- Choose a small 1-ounce pita, instead of the large 2-ounce size.
- Leave half of your turkey sandwich.
- Order a Tall cappuccino instead of a Grande next time you visit Starbucks.
- Eat one small cookie or half of a larger one.
- Buy prepackaged bags (1-ounce portions) of chips or pretzels instead of eating out of a big bag.

- Use 1 teaspoon of olive oil instead of 1 tablespoon when sautéing your vegetables. Try putting your olive oil in a spray bottle.
- Spread 1 tablespoon of peanut butter instead of 2 tablespoons on bread.
- Leave the last few bites of pasta on your plate.
- Skip bread with dinner.
- Split your favorite dessert three ways.
- Use 1 pat of butter instead of 3 pats on a baked potato.

Get the point? It doesn't really matter if you save 90 calories or 115 calories. It's the big picture that matters: *Pay attention to portions*. Here are specific activities and strategies—at home, in restaurants, in the grocery store—that bolster your portion-size awareness and give you the tools you need in every situation to downsize your diet.

smartsize your plate

Food portions are not the only thing that have increased over the years. Everything that's used to serve food and drinks—plates, bowls, glasses, tumblers, coffee cups, wine goblets, you name it—has grown in size over the past few decades. How do you deal with the upward creep of dishes? Rate your plate! Take out your serving pieces, including plates, bowls, mugs, and glasses, and take stock of the size of each container. Let's smartsize your tableware: Choose an 8- to 10-ounce glass rather than a 20-ounce tumbler; a 6- to 7-ounce wineglass rather than a 16- to 24-ounce goblet; a 9- to 10-inch-diameter dinner plate rather than a 12+-inch plate; a bowl that holds 1 to 2 cups rather than 4 to 6 cups. You don't have to get rid of your oversize serving containers—just put them away for special occasions, such as dinner parties and barbeques, and keep the smaller, more "portion-friendly"-size serving dishes and glasses in your cabinets for everyday use.

Claudette, a client of mine, had a very clever solution to supersized serving dishes. She downsized her dishes by buying a set from the 1950s at a flea market. The dishes are beautiful, but everything is much smaller. At first, she

• reality check—liquid calories •

Did you know the shape of a glass has an effect on how much you drink? University of Illinois researchers did a study showing that when given a tall, thin glass and a short, wide glass of the same size, kids at a fitness camp routinely thought they had poured less into the short, wide glass when, in reality, they had poured 77 percent more. So if you want to trick yourself into thinking you have more, use a tall, thin glass. Save your short, fat tumblers for water or seltzer.

and her family thought they were eating off toy plates, but they soon got used to it.

You can also target certain dishes, bowls, and glasses that need downsizing. I have a client who loves cereal, so much so that she used to pour herself a huge bowl, and then another, and then another . . . until she ended up eating half the huge box. Instead of downsizing her entire china service, she just exchanged her cereal "tub" for a much smaller bowl. She also switched from using a tablespoon to using a teaspoon, which forces her to eat more slowly and to savor each bite. It's awfully hard to shovel your food in when you take away the shovel.

Another client, Jean, loves ice cream. Her problem is that she has a tendency to eat the entire container (until her spoon starts scraping the bottom—oops!) or scooping it into a huge bowl and eating the whole thing. Her solution? She bought a special "ice cream bowl"—that's all she uses it for—that contains a ½-cup serving. (Jean measured it to be sure and remembered the visual of ½ baseball.) She fills this special bowl up with ice cream, eats the entire bowl, and never feels guilty. There's something about putting a ½-cup serving into a huge bowl that just shouts "deprivation." Using smaller dishes, bowls, glasses, and mugs makes less food look and feel like more.

rate your plate

To build portion awareness, try this little plating game. Measure out a standard serving size, then compare it to your normal portion. This is one of the best ways to get a mental snapshot of how much you eat and to give you a visual set point that you can measure your portion against. Here's how to practice plating.

Invest in a set of graduated measuring cups and spoons and a food scale. Get separate measuring cups for liquid and dry foods; liquids call for one type of measuring device, dry ingredients for another. The liquid measuring cup that is usually clear plastic or glass leaves some extra room so that the liquid doesn't overflow when you place it in the measuring cup. Take out your everyday plates, glasses, mugs, and bowls, the ones that you use on a daily basis.

I'm going to use cereal as an example, but you can try this procedure with anything you regularly eat and drink. To determine how much you really are eating, measure a *standard serving* of your food into your everyday dishes. (Consult the serving size chart in Appendix D.) In the case of cereal like Cheerios or bran flakes, it's 1 cup (1 baseball). Pour it in your everyday bowl. Take a mental picture of what it looks like, how far it goes up the side of the bowl, exactly how full the bowl is. Ask yourself: Is this what I usually eat, or does it look like a drop in the bucket?

Now take another bowl that's the same size as the one you just used. Pour your *typical portion* into it. Now take it out and measure it. How does it compare to a standard serving? Is it about 1 cup (or 1 standard grain serving), or is it more? My clients routinely discover that they eat two or three times the standard serving size without even realizing it. They often think "One bowl, one serving," no matter how big the bowl.

Then pour your typical portion as well as the standard serving size into smaller bowls and see how they look. A standard serving looks bigger if it's in a smaller bowl.

Use this information to adjust your portions. You may want to keep your portion large—even two to three times larger than the standard—and cut back on grains later in the day. Or you may prefer to have 1 cup of cereal at breakfast and spread out your grains during the rest of the day. Once you know how much you're eating, you can decide when and where to have your grains. If you want to cut back, try some of the smartsizing tricks in this chapter, including switching to a smaller bowl.

My client Ann tried this exercise and was shocked to find out how much peanut butter she was eating. She thought she was having only 1 tablespoon on toast, but after measuring, she found that it was closer to ½ cup. Once she was able to "eyeball" a smaller portion, it was easier to smartsize.

• portion patrol•

Help! I ate a bagel for breakfast and used up five out of six of my grains. What else can I eat for the rest of the day?

Try having a salad with protein for lunch instead of a sandwich, and for dinner opt for grilled chicken or fish with vegetables. It's okay to start with a soup. Don't have pasta as a main dish on the same day you eat a bagel in the morning. If you crave some starch at dinner, choose a high-fiber starchy vegetable like butternut squash or corn on the cob. And snack on fresh fruit and low-fat dairy instead of munching on pretzels and crackers.

smartsize your food

Does your plate runneth over? Even if you make the switch to a smaller plate, you are defeating the purpose if it's always piled high. Here are a few plating strategies to cut down on plate overflow.

1. *Put a lid on it.* Invest in plates with lids. You can purchase plastic plates that come with storage lids. After you've served yourself your meal, place the lid on top of the plate. If you can't close the lid without crushing your over-flowing food, there is too much food on your plate. If you can snap the lid on without any effort, you know you're eating a reasonable portion. You don't have to eat off these plates for good—just try the lid trick a few times to re-train your eye, and then go back to your everyday plates if you like. And take note: The only food where the lid trick isn't necessary is veggies—pile 'em on.

2. *Divide and conquer.* To eat a balanced meal, divide and conquer your plate. Draw an imaginary line down the middle of your plate, dividing it in half. Fill one half of the plate with fruits and veggies. For the other half, di-vide in half again, and fill one quarter with protein and the other quarter with starch. Try this, for example, with homemade chicken stir-fry: Fill half the plate with veggies, one quarter with chicken, and the remaining quarter with rice. If you want to skip starch at dinner, add a bit more veggies (two-thirds of the plate) and a bit more chicken (one-third of the plate), but try not to exceed one-third of the plate for the chicken or other protein-rich foods: fish, poultry, meat, beans, tofu. Note: This trick doesn't work on over-size or charger plates. Use a regular dinner plate of about 9 to 10 inches in diameter. While you are learning to get the hang of this you can purchase the plastic plates with dividers. This way you'll be sure not to load up on too much rice or pasta; you'll just put it in the small compartment.

3. *Keep portion time.* Think of your plate as a clock. Fill up half your "day" from 12 to 6 with veggies. Fill up your "evening" from 6 to 9 with protein. And fill up your "night" from 9 to 12 with starch.

smartsize a handful

Think about how often you reach into a bag of chips and grab a handful or two, then absentmindedly grab another, and another, until you've had half a jumbo bag. Do you have any idea how many chips you had, how many serving sizes your handfuls constitute, or how many servings you just ate? Whenever you eat out of large bags or containers—which I suggest you avoid—it's almost impossible to judge how many servings you're eating. Therefore, it's pretty darn hard to make any sense out of the food label and what it says about servings and nutrition.

Here's how to smartsize a handful. Food labels for snack foods, such as pretzels and chips, generally use 1-ounce servings. Take out 1 ounce of your favorite snack—say, barbeque potato chips—and measure it out. It should be around 1 cup. Look at it for a moment and take into account how much space it takes up. Put it in 2 cupped hands, getting a feel for its weight and size. Now dump the whole bag into a large serving bowl. Pick out about 1 ounce to see if you've got a feel for the serving size and how much you're grabbing. Weigh it on a food scale to see how accurate you are. If you're off, practice until you get it right (or close enough). The goal is to teach yourself to guesstimate. Then you'll have imprinted a 1-ounce serving in your mind and will never need to wonder exactly how much you're grabbing. Practice the same exercise with any other large packages or tubs of your favorite food, such as pretzels, ice cream, nuts, and so on.

think 3-d

When you're served an entrée, you may take note of how much of the plate it fills. But you also need to pay attention to the food's thickness as well as its height. Think 3-D: Take into account all dimensions of your food. Try this for baked goods, such as cookies and cakes, pancakes, and meats and fish. An extra-thick brownie or a thick steak is a bigger portion than mere length and width indicates.

speed-sizing

If your life is just too hectic to spend time plating or measuring, try instead simply to scale back one or two of your portions by either a half or a third. To scale back a sandwich, try these tricks:

- Eat only half.
- Take out a few slices of meat.
- Use only one slice of bread and make it open-face.
- Take out some of the filling and remake your own sandwich.
- Trim off what you can do without.

Choose any one of these tricks, and you're having a smaller portion, no matter the original size. No measuring, no math, no calorie counting.

smart labeling

If just eyeballing your portions isn't working for you, you may want some hard-and-fast data about how much your everyday containers hold. To learn this, take out your everyday dishes, bowls, and glasses, fill them with food, and then measure the contents. Write the amount on the bottom of one of your bowls or cups with either marking tape or a permanent marker. After you do this, you can never plead, "I had no idea just how much that bowl holds" again.

"please, sir, can i have some ... less?"

Remember the musical *Oliver?* I've edited a line from it into the heading of this section. Make it your motto. Even if you've made your home portion-control headquarters, the outside world is full of portion pressure. Here are specific strategies for any place where food is a factor: restaurants, fast-food chains, while eating and cooking at home or shopping for food. Practice a defensive outlook toward oversized food—don't buy into the consumer culture that pushes too much food on us at every turn. Defensive dining and shopping can make your motto—"Please, sir, can I have some . . . less?"—easy to put into practice.

smartsize your restaurant meal

Let me share a story about Kara, a client of mine in her mid-forties, who moved from England to the United States. When she came here and started eating at restaurants, she left some food on her plate; she was, after all, used

portion shockers . . .

- Nearly 50 percent of every food dollar is spent on foods and meals away from home according to USDA.
- The Lone Star Café features the sirloin steak challenge, a 72-ounce steak, "which separates the men from the boys," and is free if you can finish it, along with its trimmings, in less than one hour. This is nine full days' worth of meat.
- A 64-ounce "Mega-rita" is a margarita that can fill a half gallon (2 quarts).
- Claim Jumper, a chain based in California, has made a name for itself in the marketplace with its mammoth offerings, including the famous Six Layer Chocolate Motherlode Cake, which costs $7.95 a slice and is big enough to feed an entire family.

to smaller portions. The waitstaff asked her, "Was the food okay?" and she sheepishly nodded, thinking she was hurting their feelings. Rather than go through the trouble with the waitstaff, Kara started finishing everything on her plate and quickly put on fifteen pounds. Remember, you *don't* have to finish your plate when dining at a restaurant. In fact, you should not finish it, especially when a portion for one is really enough food to serve two or three.

- Steer clear of buffets and all-you-can-eat deals.
- Don't go to the restaurant feeling famished. Eat a small snack before you go.
- Skip the bread basket, especially if you want some starch with your entrée.
- Order appetizer or "half-size" portions.
- Order small instead of large orders.
- Steer clear of ordering dishes that include the words "large," "giant," and "jumbo."
- Order a doggie bag *before* your meal: When your food arrives, eyeball your appropriate portion, and ask the waitstaff to wrap up the rest before you begin your meal. A doggie bag makes a great accessory!
- Order salad dressing and sauces on the side. That way, you can see exactly how much you're pouring on.
- Skip the starch entirely, and get double veggies.
- Start your meal with vegetable-based soups or salad.
- Share a main-dish entrée.
- When splitting entrées, order an extra salad or extra veggies.
- Share a sandwich and order a salad or a side of veggies.
- Top your sandwich with greens, carrots, or tomatoes.
- At a steakhouse, order the smallest beef entrée portion—even that size is large.
- Split the baked potato if it's jumbo size.
- Guesstimate your portions with your palm, not your purse.
- Eat half of whatever you order—you'll be eating the same amount as restaurant-goers did twenty years ago.
- Euro-size it! Eat like a Parisian or a Roman where portions are smaller and people eat less.

- Don't inhale your food, chew it. Put your fork down between bites.
- Don't measure your dining experience by the size of your portion. Enjoy the experience, including the taste, company, and surroundings.
- Give up your membership in the clean-plate club. It's okay not to finish your meal.
- Pay attention to your Hunger Meter: Stop when you're comfortable, not when you're stuffed. Wrap up leftovers.
- Remember, this is not your "last supper."

• reality check—jumbo sizes •

No matter what it is—pet food, plant food, candy, chips, and even non-food items—research shows that you will pour more out of a jumbo package. Period. That's a good reason to steer clear of anything jumbo if you don't want to wear jumbo sizes.

• portion patrol •

Help! I know that I should try to avoid buffets and all-you-can-eat deals, but I love to frequent such places. Any suggestions for surviving while at a buffet?

Here are a few smartsizing tips while eating at a buffet. Preplan. Before loading food onto your plate, take a stroll down the entire buffet line to find out the choices available to you. Think about the foods that you would really enjoy and fit them into your plan. Pass on the foods that don't really move you. The good news about a buffet is that often you can get healthy choices. Fill up on fresh veggies, fruits, and salads with dressings on the side. Skip foods with lots of sauces and dressings. Take one decent-size plate and don't go back for more. Limit the tastes and nibbles. Eat only what you put on your plate, and eat only while sitting and engaging in conversation. And remember, eat slowly, savor each bite, and enjoy your company. And, to be certain you don't overeat, do not wear loose-fitting clothes to the buffet.

smartsize your fast-food meal

Even a passing glance at the size-inflation timelines in the first chapter and in Appendix F shows how fast-food restaurants, in particular, have supersized everything on their menu. No matter the label or description a fast-food place attaches to any menu offering, it's probably still too large. Just because a fast-food restaurant calls its fries or soda medium doesn't mean that it's an acceptable amount to eat or drink. Research shows that the actual amount we are served is a lot larger than it was in the past, even if the label description, such as medium, is the same. That's why you should get kiddie or small sizes at all fast-food chains. If it's too difficult for you to go from king to kiddie immediately, smartsize down one portion size at a time. Make the switch from large to medium and then, next time, from medium to small. And one day, graduate to kiddie size, which is totally acceptable, if not preferable, even for adults. Here are some additional tips:

- Order small sizes instead of large sizes, mini instead of mammoth.
- Order single instead of double or triple burgers; quarter-pounder instead of half-pounder.
- Steer clear of words like "biggie," "extra large," "king," "upsize," "super-size," "roundup," "jumbo," and "mega." They all mean more food, which always means more calories.

• reality check—bunless burger •

What's the story with the bunless burgers? Are they the way to go? No! Instead of a thick burger *without* a bun, you are better off with a thin burger (a smaller burger) with a bun. Believe it or not, the thin burger and bun has fewer calories. It is pointless to deprive yourself of bread when you're going overboard on a jumbo burger that's filled with fat and calories. (That's a bit like ordering a diet soda with a huge meal with all the trimmings and dessert.) It's all about balance: It's better to cut your big burger in half, and eat that, rather than just removing the bread.

• reality check—low-carb pizza •

With all of the advertising out there on low-carb foods, are low-carb choices any lower in calories and is purchasing low-carb alternatives the way to go? Absolutely not! Indulging in a small slice of pizza on occasion is better than going low-carb and having several slices because you think it is "diet food." In a study I conducted with the staff of *People* magazine, we found that ounce for ounce, a low-carb pizza slice actually had more calories than a regular pizza slice.

smartsize your supermarket shopping

portion shockers . . .

- In 1988 the original Lunchables was small and contained 340 calories. By the year 2000, Oscar Mayer introduced the Lunchables Mega Pack, containing 640 calories for the pizza version and 780 calories for nacho version.
- When Thomas' English Muffins introduced Sandwich Size English muffins, which are 65 percent larger than their regular size, sales went up 2,500 percent.
- When Lender's introduced the Big 'N Crusty frozen bagels, sales increased 68 percent.
- The original Kellogg's Raisin Bran box in 1942 was 15 ounces. Today the jumbo box is 25.5 ounces.
- Swanson's All Day Breakfast, a new frozen meal in the Hungry-Man line, is over a pound and contains *all* of the following: eggs, pancakes, hash browns, sausage, and bacon.
- Swanson's Hungry-Man XXL dinners rang up or generated $17.8 million in 2003.

It all starts here. If you don't buy big packages for your home, you won't eat them. Now, more than ever, jumbo-size food packaging is stuffing the aisles of your local supermarket. Here's the smartsize guide to supermarkets.

- In supermarket aisles, avoid jumbo bags and boxes of food. It's okay to buy bulk paper towels—you don't eat them and they don't get stale.
- Jumbo-size packages may save you a dollar here or there, but they are no health bargain.

- Buy single-serving portions whenever possible. They may cost more, but your health and well-being are worth it.
- Beware of tiny snacks, such as bite-size crackers and cookies. Their size is deceptive, often luring you into a nibble here, a nibble there, until you've eaten much more than you realize.
- If you know you're the type who eats ice cream by the carton (you learned it when analyzing your Portion Personality), buy frozen pops, ice cream sandwiches, or other single-serve items instead.
- Read food labels. Check for the number of servings per container. You may be surprised.
- Bulk up on fresh fruits and veggies.
- Load your cart with healthful choices before going to the bakery, candy, and snack aisles.
- Don't go to the supermarket when you're hungry.

• portion patrol •

Help! What's the deal with store-bought single-serving entrées? Can I have them for dinner sometimes?

Prepackaged meals are okay occasionally, but don't get in the habit of eating them regularly. Many of these items are high in sodium, so if you're going to have one, be sure to check the food label and watch your salt intake throughout the day. Stick with the healthier choices—baked chicken instead of fried. The good news about Lean Cuisines and the like are that they are portion-controlled—that's why they are low in calories and can help people lose weight. These meals can help you to retrain your eye on what a reasonable portion looks like. Same with meals like the Zone delivery—they are portion-controlled and taste good. Feel free to add a large salad and lots of steamed veggies if you'd like. Remember, as long as you don't glob on lots of dressing and sauce, you can bulk up your meal with vegetables.

• reality check—single serving •

Sara was chowing down every morning on the new single-serve Super Size Raisin Bran Crunch cereal in a cup, thinking that was a healthy way to start the day. Little did she know that it has nearly 300 calories and is 3 grain servings, even though it's marketed as a "single-serve" item. Watch out for all oversize single-serve portions that are clearly jumbo size. You need to judge for yourself and create your own single-serve: eat half! And be on the lookout for 1-ounce single servings: They truly are for one person.

smartsize your home

We've become so accustomed to bigger portions in restaurants that they've crept into our homes as well. We eat off big dishes, we cook from books that suggest larger portions, and we believe that we must finish our food "because there are children starving in other parts of the world." It's important to pay attention to the messages that we receive in our own homes to eat more. With a few simple tricks and tips, you can make small but effective changes at home.

- Smartsize your plates, glasses, mugs, and utensils.
- Use an appetizer plate or a bread plate for your main dish.
- Use a teaspoon instead of a tablespoon; use a salad fork instead of an entrée fork.
- Don't eat while at the stove or preparing food in the kitchen.
- Don't eat directly from fridge/freezer. Sit down, set the table, and enjoy your meal or snack.

- Don't eat directly out of the bag or container. Plate it so you're forced to see how much you're eating.
- At the end of your family meal, wrap up leftovers immediately. Use small plastic containers for storing single-serve portions.
- Avoid serving food "family style."
- Follow the rule of one. Whatever you're eating, with the exception of vegetables, have only one helping: one chicken breast, one helping of rice, one sliver of cake.
- When cooking more than one meal or serving, freeze foods that you are not planning to eat immediately in single-serve portions.
- Bag it! Once you open a bag of nibble food such as pretzels or chips, portion it out into single servings and put it in zip-lock bags. If the label says 10 servings per container, use 10 bags.
- Don't keep food out on the counter.
- Store sweets and treats in opaque storage containers. If you can't see them, you won't be as tempted.
- Close the bag. An open bag screams "Eat me!"
- Learn to cook. Measuring out ingredients gives you a feel for food size.
- Halve your recipes. If you prepare half as much, you can eat only half as much.
- Make casseroles in individual-size baking dishes so you won't be tempted to overeat.
- Use mini-muffin tins instead of jumbo tins. You may even want to try muffin top tins. (Yes, they are available, and they are easy to find.)
- Read food labels. Compare how much *you* actually eat to the serving sizes on the food label.
- Eat slowly. Savor each bite.
- Wait fifteen minutes before you go back for seconds.
- Put your fork down in between bites. Or try chopsticks.
- Eat your fruit instead of drinking it—keep fresh fruit on hand instead of juices. If you must have juice, try diluting it with water.
- When in doubt, leave it out.

• reality check—see food •

At a work site study, people ate nine candies per person when chocolate was visible on their desk, six candies when the candy was in the desk drawer, and only three when the candies were out of sight. The clear message? The more you see, the more you eat. My clients Larry and Caroline made a few small changes in their home—they put away the snack and candy jar and tucked food into the cabinet—and found that they immediately ate less.

favorite-food makeover

Ask yourself this question: What's my favorite food? Whatever your answer, there's a good chance that its average portion is too large. Many people eat too much of the same foods over and over again: pasta, meat entrées, bagels, and muffins. Let's zero in on some of your favorite foods and determine how to move from hefty portions to smartsize portions.

FOOD/PORTION	HEFTY PORTION	SMARTSIZE PORTION
BAGEL	5–7 ounces (giant size)	2–3 ounces (1/2 bagel or scooped out bagel)
MUFFIN	6–8 ounces (large size)	Muffin top (3 ounces)
CHOCOLATE BAR	2 1/2–5 ounces (king-giant size)	1 ounce (4 squares)
COOKIE	4 ounces (single serving)	1/2–1 ounce (1-Oreo-size)
STEAK	24 ounces (restaurant entrée)	4 ounces (1 1/2 decks of cards)
CHICKEN/FISH ENTRÉE	7–8 ounces (restaurant entrée)	4 ounces (1 1/2 decks of cards)
PASTA	3 cups (restaurant entrée)	1 1/2 cups (1 1/2 baseballs) (appetizer portion)
RICE	1 pint/2 cups (Chinese takeout)	1 cup (1 baseball)
PIZZA BY THE SLICE	14–16 ounces (2 slices with extra cheese)	5–7 ounces (1 regular slice)
POPCORN	16 cups (medium at theater)	3 cups (3 baseballs)
PRETZELS	6 ounces (hot pretzel from street vendor)	1-ounce bag
SANDWICH FILLING: *Roast beef/turkey/ tuna*	6–8 ounces (local deli)	3–4 ounces (1/2 sandwich or 1 1/2 decks of cards)
SODA (FOUNTAIN)	64 fl ounces (Double Gulp)	8 fl ounces (1 cup or 1/2 Gulp)
SODA (FAST-FOOD)	32 fl ounces (large)	12 fl ounces (child size)
SODA BOTTLE	20 fl ounces (vending machine size)	8-ounce bottle
BEER	24 fl ounces (large can)	12-ounce can
ORANGE JUICE	16 fl ounces (pint)	7-ounce bottle

Here's another way of looking at smartsizing in action. Switching from Living Large to Living Lean saves you lots of servings:

LIVING LARGE	LIVING LEAN	SERVINGS SAVED
PASTA ENTRÉE (6 grains)	PASTA APPETIZER (3 grain)	3 grain
STREET PRETZEL (6 grains)	SMALL BAG (1 grain)	5 grain
BAGEL (5 grains)	ENGLISH MUFFIN (2 grain)	3 grain
MUFFIN (6½ grains)	WHOLE-GRAIN WAFFLE (1 grain)	5½ grain
24 OUNCES/ 18 OUNCES COOKED PORTERHOUSE (6 meats)	9 OUNCES/6 OUNCES COOKED SIRLOIN (2 meat)	4 meat
PINT OF OJ (almost 3 fruits)	1 ORANGE (1 fruit)	Almost 2 fruit

smartsize your favorite foods

SMARTSIZE PASTA

Standard Portion Teller Serving Size:	½ cup cooked pasta	=	1 grain serving	= ½ baseball
Typical Restaurant Servings:				
Main dish portions	3 cups cooked pasta	=	6 grain servings	= 3 baseballs
Appetizer portions	1 ½ cups cooked pasta	=	3 grain servings	= 1 ½ baseballs

Restaurant Survival Tips

- Order an appetizer portion or a half portion.
- Share an entrée with your dining companion.
- Order pasta with lots of vegetables.
- If you plan to eat pasta for dinner, watch your bread intake throughout the day. Limit bagels and muffins at breakfast. Choose low-fat dairy, fruits, vegetables, fish, or poultry earlier in the day. And especially steer clear of the bread at the dinner table.
- Order a tossed salad or share an appetizer to avoid eating from the bread basket.
- Eat half of what you are served and ask the waiter to wrap the rest up. It's best to do that as soon as it arrives, so you won't be tempted.
- Pay attention to the size of your bowl or plate. Bigger plates hold more food.
- Stop eating when you are full, regardless of how much is left on your plate.
- Note: One pasta entrée is practically an entire day's worth of grain, so go easy.

• portion patrol•

Help! I am going out to dinner tonight, and I know I'll be eating a lot later. What can I snack on *now*?

If you deprive yourself during the day, you'll just end up overeating later. Instead, have an appetizer-type snack in the late afternoon. Then skip the appetizer at the restaurant. A few good late-afternoon snacks are: vegetable, minestrone, or bean soup; a tossed salad or spinach salad; mixed veggies or pita dipped in hummus; a slice of cheese on whole-wheat toast; fresh fruit and yogurt; a glass of V8 juice and 3 Kavli Crisp breads; 3 whole-grain breadsticks; or a baked sweet potato with nonfat sour cream.

Home Survival Tips

- Learn to recognize what a serving looks like. Read the serving size information on the Nutrition Facts label. Be sure to note how many servings are in the entire package and how many servings you are actually cooking and eating.
- Measure out your portion. This will help you eyeball your portion when eating out. To fix the proper size in your mind, you just need to measure your portion a few times.
- Eat on a smaller plate; your portion will look bigger.
- Prepare a smaller portion of pasta. Mix it with a marinara sauce and lots of vegetables. And start your meal with a nice salad instead of bread.
- Avoid serving pasta "family style." Plate out portions in advance, and avoid seconds.

SMARTSIZE TUNA, TURKEY, CHICKEN, OR ROAST BEEF SANDWICH (FILLING ONLY)

Standard Portion Teller Serving Size: 3 ounces cooked fish, poultry, or meat = 1 meat serving (deck of cards)
Typical Sandwich Filling: 6 ounces = 2 meat servings (2 decks of cards)

Restaurant Survival Tips

- Order a half sandwich and a salad.
- Share a sandwich with your dining companion.
- If you eat a typical sandwich for lunch, watch your meat intake throughout the day. Choose beans, low-fat dairy, fruits, and vegetables. For dinner, try for rice and beans.
- Make your own sandwich: Order 4 ounces or a "quarter pound" of tuna (turkey, etc.), 2 slices of bread, and include a tossed salad or a mixed vegetable platter.

- Eat half of what you are served and wrap the rest up for tomorrow.
- Note: One store-bought sandwich is often an entire day's worth of meat!!

Home Survival Tips

- Learn to recognize what a serving looks like. Read the serving size information on the Nutrition Facts label. For example, use a 3-ounce individual can of tuna or half a 6-ounce can.
- Portion out (and wrap up) turkey and deli meats in 3- to 4-ounce portions and store in your refrigerator.
- Cut your sandwich into quarters.

SMARTSIZE MUFFIN

Standard Portion Teller serving size: 1-ounce muffin = 1 grain serving (a bite-size mini muffin or about ⅙ of a muffin)
Typical Size: 6½ ounces = 6½ grain servings

Survival Tips

- If you eat a muffin for breakfast, watch your bread intake throughout the day. Limit pasta and rice. Choose low-fat dairy, fruits, vegetables, fish, or poultry throughout the day. And especially steer clear of the bread at the dinner table.
- Have ½ muffin, a "mini" muffin, or a muffin top instead of an entire jumbo muffin. Add some low-fat dairy and fruit.
- Try having a high-fiber breakfast cereal or 2 slices whole-grain bread instead of the muffin.
- Note: A muffin contains an entire day's worth of grains.

SMARTSIZE BAGEL

Standard Portion Teller Serving Size: 1-ounce bagel = 1 grain serving (½ yo-yo)
Typical Size: 5 ounces = 5 bread servings

Survival Tips

- If you eat a bagel for breakfast, watch your bread intake throughout the day. Limit pasta and rice. Choose low-fat dairy, fruits, vegetables, fish, or poultry throughout the day. And especially steer clear of the bread at the dinner table.
- Have ½ bagel instead of an entire bagel. Add some low-fat dairy and fruit instead of cream cheese or butter.
- Scoop out your bagel. A scooped-out bagel is about 3 grain servings instead of 5 servings.
- Try having a sandwich on whole-wheat bread instead of a bagel. You'll get lots more fiber and you will save calories.
- Note: One bagel contains practically an entire day's worth of grain.

pump up the volume

Throughout this chapter, you've learned many different ways to cut down on your portions, to smartsize instead of supersize. Well, what if you're tired of eating less? What if eating less doesn't really work for you and is one of the main reasons you never seem to lose weight? You don't want to feel deprived. Well, here is a solution: Pump up the volume! It's okay to add volume to your diet, as long as you know which foods add bulk without adding too many calories. Barbara Rolls and colleagues at Pennsylvania State University discovered how to eat more food without more calories. The key is to fill up on more water-rich foods. Increase fresh veggies, fruits, and veggie-based soups. Top sandwiches with salad greens, have ½ sandwich plus a nice-size salad for lunch, add baby carrots as a snack, top your cereal or yogurt with berries or sliced bananas, enjoy a fresh fruit salad as an afternoon snack. At a restaurant, order fresh berries and a cappuccino made from skim milk for dessert and allow yourself a few bites of your dinner companion's dessert. If you have the fruit, you won't feel deprived and won't need more than just two bites of dessert as a taste. Start your dinner with a tossed salad or a veggie-based soup, especially in a restaurant. By doing so, you will be less likely to eat from the bread basket.

Carolyn, a woman in her mid-fifties, was overeating grains because she was skimping on fruits and veggies. By pumping up the volume and incorporating more fruits and veggies into her diet, she was more satisfied. Instead of a bowl of cereal plus 2 pieces of rye toast at breakfast, she added a fruit salad and was able to skip the toast. She also included more vegetable soups and salads at lunch and dinner and was able to do without her usual roll and mashed potatoes.

portion shocker . . .

If you want to eat less, add a little air! Pennsylvania State University researchers examined appetites of men given milk shakes whipped to varying degrees of frothiness. They found that those who had milkshakes whipped up twice as much ate 12 percent less.

• reality check—salad •

Pennsylvania State University researchers found that people who started their lunch with a large low-fat salad ate 12 percent fewer calories during that meal. The same goes for soup before a meal. Eat more and lose weight! How's that for a dieter's dream? But salad lovers beware: Skip the croutons and cheese and order a low-fat dressing, or be sure to get the salad dressing on the side.

• get smart! •

Make these simple substitutions, and you will be eating the same amount in terms of servings per food group, but you get a lot more food for a similar nutrient value. In other words, a lot more volume in each serving—not a bad deal!

- Switch from 1 serving of pretzels (¾ cup or 1 tennis ball) to 1 serving of popcorn (3 cups or 3 baseballs).
- Switch from 1 serving of meat (3 ounces or 1 deck of cards) to the equivalent of a meat alternative such as lentils (1 cup or 1 baseball).
- Switch from 1 serving of cheese (1½ ounces or 6 dice) to 1 serving yogurt (one 8-ounce container).
- Switch from 1 serving of bread (1 slice) to 1 serving mini rice cakes (5 rice cakes).
- Switch from 1 serving of juice (6 ounces) to 1 serving of cantaloupe (1 cup).
- Switch from 1 serving of dried fruit (¼ cup or 1 golf ball) to 1 serving of berries (1 cup or 1 baseball).

Puff it up! Go from the same amount of a calorically dense food to the same amount of a less calorically dense food from the same food group, and look at how many servings you'll save:

- Switch from 1 cup granola or 1 baseball (4 grain) to 1 cup or 1 baseball puffed wheat (½ grain). Save 3½ grain.
- Switch from 1 cup or 1 baseball pretzels (1¼ grain) to 1 cup or 1 baseball popcorn (⅓ grain) and save almost 1 grain.
- Switch from 1 cup or 1 baseball raisins (4 fruit) to 1 cup or 1 baseball grapes (1 fruit) and save 3 fruit.
- Substitute a smart bet: Swap whole milk for fat-free milk and save lots of fat. Swap red meat for fish or poultry. Swap a hamburger for a veggie burger.

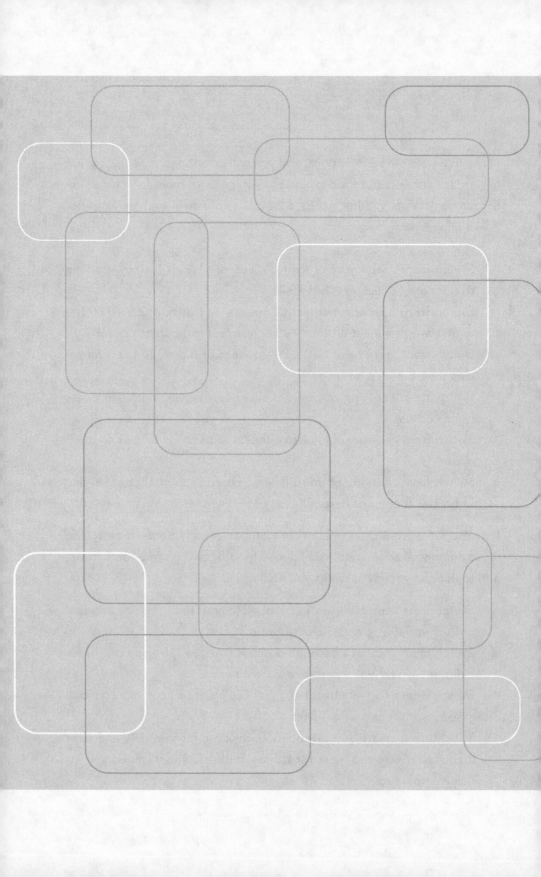

epilogue

"How long does getting thin take?"
Pooh asked anxiously.
• A. A. MILNE, *WINNIE-THE-POOH*

There are many ways to measure "success" on a food plan, the first of which is weight loss. But it's not the only measure of success, and certainly not the only goal of *The Portion Teller*. How many of you can say that, before you learned how to smartsize, you looked at a meat entrée or a plate of pasta and thought to yourself, "I wonder how many carbs are in that? Is it loaded with fat? And what about the calories?" It's my hope that these questions have faded away, and, instead, you say to yourself: "How big is this portion? How does it compare to a deck of cards or a baseball? And how does it fit into my eating plan for today?" In my experience, a fresh, portion-size outlook, one that takes into account how much you eat and incorporates it into an ongoing effort to eat well and balance your portions, is the best measure of success. I've seen people throw away all the numbers, charts, percentages, and fads, only to find that a new outlook often goes hand in hand with weight loss. It's almost miraculous; I can't tell you the number of people who tell me how easy, fun, simple, and effective smartsizing is, all without the kind of negative, restricted time period "on" a diet.

Without a period of time "on" or "off," you may wonder how you should measure your own progress. I don't ask clients to stick to a certain regimen for one week and then switch to another, nor do I tell them they can start to integrate new foods into their eating plan once they've reached certain "levels." And since there's no going "on," there's no going "off." Instead, smart-sizing is forever. I've found that once people know how much they're eating, they can't eat with abandon anymore—information ruins their ability to say, "I had no idea I was eating so much." With the Portion Teller plan, your awareness will get in the way of both *under*estimating your portions and *over*eating whatever you're served.

I have tried to introduce the information in *The Portion Teller* so that you can build on it, learning the separate concepts slowly, so that you can incorporate them into your lifestyle. The real work begins with visuals. I suggest you spend at least a week or two training yourself to use the visual comparisons and the Handy Method. It doesn't take much time or effort to look at everything you eat and consider exactly how big it is in comparison to the visuals. No one needs to know you're even doing it, especially when you are looking at your own palm or thumb. (That isn't the case if you pull out a scale or calculator at the dinner table.)

After you have a basic understanding of the size of your foods, it's time to examine your diet, determine your Portion Personality, and keep the Portion Teller Diary. You may use the diary as long as you see fit, but I recommend that you keep track of your eating habits for a minimum of a month. Some of my clients continue to use it over time to chart their progress and to see exactly which eating habits lead to weight loss and feeling energetic and healthy. But you don't have to keep up the Portion Teller Diary forever; you can graduate to the Portion Teller Progress Sheet.

Once you know your own habits, you graduate to food substitutions. Here you hone your ability to make simple substitutions within each food group, switching from, say, a pasta entrée (6 grains) to a grilled chicken breast with a side of rice (2 grains), saving 4 grain servings. Again, I suggest you spend some time getting used to thinking of your food in a new way; instead of seeing a bagel, you'll see a whole day's worth of grains, perhaps spread out over the day at each meal. After a while, you'll be a natural Portion Teller. You won't need to write anything down or keep track of your food groups and servings; portion awareness will become second nature, a part of your life, just like exercise or your favorite hobby, something you know so well that you don't have to spend too much time thinking about it. It's how you live. Now, that's what I call success. But if you need more material gains—or, in this case, losses—I suggest you keep track of your weight by weighing yourself once or twice a week. (Any more than that is too much and doesn't take into account water weight or temporary fluctuations.) Or you can use my preferred method: Choose a pair of pants to track your progress. You know which pair of jeans is a little tight and exactly where they're snug. Slip them on once a week and get a sense of how they fit. Don't expect them to fall off you in a month; this is a permanent program, not a crash diet, so success is measured over the long haul.

Which brings me to the last point I want to make: There is no such thing as a Portion Teller failure. Any Portion Teller knows: You can't change the past, only the future. There's always another day to practice awareness and to make even the smallest of changes. It may be just a smaller glass of juice. Or perhaps a decision to break off half of a cookie, eating half now and saving the rest for later. Or to take a slice of turkey out of your sandwich. In each case, you've made progress—portion progress—and that's always a success.

Test what you've learned about portions
with the Wheel of Portion quiz

1. A typical deli/bakery bagel is equal to approximately _____ slices of bread (and servings of grains).
a. 2
b. 3
c. 5
d. 8
correct answer: c

2. A take-out order of your favorite Chinese food comes with a side of rice. How many cups does that portion of rice contain?
a. ½ cup
b. 1 cup
c. 2 cups
d. 3 cups
correct answer: c

3. How many standard grain servings are in that side of rice?
a. 1
b. 2
c. 3
d. 4
correct answer: d

4. A ½-cup serving of cooked rice looks like:

a. a golf ball

b. ½ baseball

c. a baseball

d. a walnut

correct answer: b

5. All of the following are ways to cut down your intake of meat while dining in a restaurant except:

a. sharing a meat entrée with a friend

b. ordering an extra portion of sides dishes, such as vegetables and baked potato

c. just ordering off the menu

d. ordering two entrées—one meat entrée and one vegetarian entrée—and a large salad and splitting them several ways

correct answer: c

6. For lunch, Jane ate a turkey sandwich (3 ounces turkey on 2 slices rye bread), a cup of vegetable soup, and an apple. Her lunch included . . .

a. 1 serving from the grain group, 1 serving from the meat group, 1 serving from the vegetable group, and 1 serving from the fruit group

b. 2 servings from the grain group, 1 serving from the meat group, 1 serving from the vegetable group, and 1 serving from the fruit group

c. 3 servings from the grain group, 2 servings from the meat group, 1 serving from the vegetable group, and 1 serving from the fruit group

d. 2 servings from the grain group, 2 servings from the meat group, 2 servings from the vegetable group, and 1 serving from the fruit group

correct answer: b

7. A 1-ounce serving of ready-to-eat (cold) cereal translates into approximately:

a. 1 baseball or 1 cup Cheerios

b. 1 golf ball or ¼ cup granola

c. 2 baseballs or 2 cups puffed rice

d. all of the above

correct answer: d

8. A pint of orange juice contains _____ ounces.

a. 4

b. 8

c. 12

d. 16

correct answer: d

9. Your friend drank a pint of orange juice for breakfast. This translates into how many fruit servings?

a. 1; after all, it is 1 pint

b. 2

c. almost 3

d. 4

correct answer: c

10. Which vegetable(s) are counted as a grain/starch serving on this program?

a. corn

b. peas

c. baked potato

d. all of the above

correct answer: d

11. One serving of fruit is equal to:

a. 6 ounces juice

b. 1 piece of fruit

c. 1 cup berries

d. all of the above

correct answer: d

12. All of the following contain the same number of grain servings except:

a. bran muffin

b. bialy

c. English muffin

d. hamburger roll

correct answer: a

13. All of the following are meat alternatives and equivalent to 1 ounce of meat except:

a. ½ cup beans

b. ½ cup tofu

c. 2 ounces cheese

d. 1 egg

correct answer: c

14. Which of the following is an incorrect standard serving size according to The Portion Teller?

a. ½ baseball or ½ cup rice

b. deck of cards or 3 ounces chicken

c. one 8-ounce yogurt container or 1 glass milk

d. 1 baseball or 1 cup nuts

correct answer: d

15. A hot pretzel from a street vendor is equivalent to:

a. 6 bread slices

b. 6 small bags (1 ounce) pretzels

c. 18 cups popcorn

d. all of the above

correct answer: d

16. A medium popcorn at the movie theater contains:

a. 4 cups

b. 7 cups

c. 12 cups

d. 16 cups

correct answer: d

17. Approximately how many standard grain servings does this popcorn translate into?

a. 2

b. 5

c. 8

d. 1; it's only one bucket

correct answer: b

18. According to The Portion Teller, nuts and nut butters falls into which category?

a. treats and sweets

b. fats

c. grains and starchy vegetables

d. meats and meat alternatives

correct answer: b

19. You hear that nuts contain a healthy fat. A standard size translates into:

a. a fist's worth

b. 1 level hand

c. 2 cupped handfuls

d. 1 handful

correct answer: b

20. A single-serve muffin weighs, on average:

a. 1.5 ounces

b. 2 ounces

c. 4 ounces

d. 6.5 ounces

correct answer: d

21. A standard serving of beer is 12 ounces. You purchase and drink one 24-ounce can. How many servings is that?

a. 1; it's one can and one portion

b. 1.5

c. 2

d. 3

correct answer: c

22. You are at a cocktail party and can't resist the cheese cubes. How much cheese translates into 1 dairy serving?

a. 2 dice or ½ ounce

b. 6 to 8 dice or 1½ to 2 ounces

c. 12 dice or 3 ounces

d. 16 dice or 4 ounces

correct answer: b

23. How many ounces of soda were in the individual single-serving size bottle of Coca-Cola at the time of the first Apollo lunar mission?

a. 6.5 ounce

b. 8 ounces

c. 12 ounces

d. 16 ounces

correct answer: a

24. Which size soda bottle is currently found in a vending machine?

a. 6.5 ounces

b. 8 ounces

c. 16 ounces

d. 20 ounces

correct answer: d

25. The original size Hershey bar in 1908 weighed how many ounces?

a. 0.6 ounces, and the size of today's "fun bar"

b. 1 ounce

c. 1.6 ounce, the size of a standard bar

d. 2 ounces

correct answer: a

26. Many steaks at a steakhouse are 24 ounces (18 ounces cooked) and contain how many meat servings?

a. 3, 1 day's worth

b. 4

c. 6, at least 2 days' worth

d. 10

correct answer: c

27. You purchase a healthy looking soup that you think contains 1 serving. The label says that each serving contains 100 calories and that there are 2½ servings per container. Of course, you eat the whole thing. How many calories did you consume?

a. 100 calories

b. 150

c. 200

d. 250

correct answer: d

28. One egg is equal to how many ounces of meat?

a. 1

b. 2

c. 3

d. 4

correct answer: a

29. *What is a standard serving size for cooked pasta according to* The Portion Teller?

a. 1 golf ball or ¼ cup

b. ½ baseball or ½ cup

c. 1 baseball or 1 cup

d. 2 baseballs or 2 cups

correct answer: b

30. *How many standard servings does a typical restaurant entrée contain?*

a. 2

b. 4

c. 6

d. 8

correct answer: c

31. *You love salad but know that salad dressing can be fattening. You are trying to aim for 1 tablespoon of dressing for your salad. What does that look like?*

a. 1 thumb tip

b. 3 thumb tips

c. 1 finger

d. none of the above

correct answer: b

32. *According to the Portion Teller Pyramid, French fries fall into which category?*

a. vegetable

b. treats and sweets

c. grains and starchy vegetable

d. none of the above

correct answer: b

33. One grain serving of popcorn is 3 cups, or which of the following?

a. 3 tight fists

b. 3 baseballs

c. 3 golf balls

d. a and b

correct answer: d

34. One hot pretzel from a street vendor translates into how many grain servings?

a. 1

b. 3

c. 6

d. 8

correct answer: c

35. All of the following are 2-grain servings and can be substituted for one another except:

a. 1 baseball or 1 cup couscous

b. 2 golf balls or ½ baseball or ½ cup granola

c. 4 baseballs or 4 cups puffed wheat cereal

d. ½ baseball or ½ cup Cheerios

correct answer: d

36. A deck of cards is approximately how many ounces of meat?

a. 1

b. 3

c. 5

d. none of the above

correct answer: b

measuring up

portion equivalents/ conversion chart

In love, as in gluttony, pleasure is a matter of the utmost precision.

• ITALO CALVINO

Volume Measurements

Fluid Ounces	Cups	Tablespoons
1	⅛	2
2	¼	4 (restaurant portion of salad dressing)
4	½	8
8	1	16

1 pint = 16 fluid ounces = 2 cups   (kiddie movie soda)

1 quart = 32 fluid ounces = 2 pints = 4 cups   (large soda at McDonald's)

½ gallon = 64 fluid ounces = 2 quarts = 4 pints = 8 cups   (7-Eleven Double Gulp)

1 gallon = 128 fluid ounces = 4 quarts = 8 pints = 16 cups

Conversions: U.S. to Metric (slightly rounded)

U.S. Volume Measure	Metric
¼ teaspoon	1 milliliter
½ teaspoon	2 milliliters
1 teaspoon	5 milliliters
1 tablespoon, ½ fluid ounce	15 milliliters
2 tablespoons, 1 fluid ounce	30 milliliters
¼ cup, 2 fluid ounces	60 milliliters
½ cup, 4 fluid ounces	120 milliliters
¾ cup, 6 fluid ounces	180 milliliters
1 cup, 8 fluid ounces	240 milliliters
1 quart, 32 fluid ounces	950 milliliters
1 quart + 3 tablespoons	1 liter
1 gallon, 128 fluid ounces	4 liters

Note: 1 tablespoon = 3 teaspoons

1 liter = 1,000 milliliters

Weight Measurements

Conversion: U.S. to Metric (slightly rounded)

1 ounce = 28.4 grams (approximately 28 to 30 grams)

Ounces	Grams
1	30
2	60
3.5	100
4	115 (4 ounces = ¼ pound)
6	170
8	230
12	340 (12 ounces = ¾ pound)
16	455 (16 ounces = 1 pound)

other useful portion teller
measurement tips

One cup does not equal 8 ounces when it comes to solids. One cup equals 8 ounces only for liquids. Cereal is a good example of this.

1 ounce ready-to-eat (cold) cereal =

> 2 cups puffed wheat or puffed rice
>
> 1 cup rice cereal
>
> 1 cup oat rings (Cheerios)
>
> 1 cup cereal flakes (Total)
>
> ½ cup Shredded Wheat (spoon size)
>
> ¼ cup granola
>
> ¼ cup nuggets (Grape-Nuts)

Food Yields

1 ounce uncooked pasta = ½ cup cooked

2 ounces uncooked pasta = 1 cup cooked

8 ounces uncooked spaghetti = 4 cups cooked

1 cup dry macaroni = 2 cups cooked

3 tablespoons uncooked rice = ½ cup cooked

1 cup uncooked rice = approximately 4 cups cooked

½ cup popcorn kernels = approximately 4 cups popped

½ cup uncooked oatmeal = 1 cup cooked

4 ounces uncooked chicken, fish, or beef = approximately 3 ounces cooked

8 ounces uncooked chicken, fish, or beef = approximately 6 ounces cooked

• appendix b •

portion teller diary

FOOD (INCLUDE METHOD OF PREPARATION)	YOUR PORTION	FOOD GROUP	NUMBER OF SERVINGS

BREAKFAST:

LUNCH:

SNACK:

DINNER:

SNACK:

FRUITS:

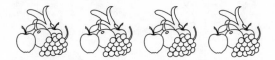

VEGETABLES:

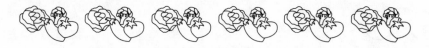

GRAINS AND STARCHY VEGETABLES:

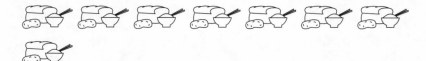

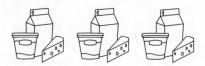

DAIRY:

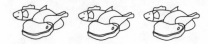

FISH, POULTRY, MEATS, AND MEAT ALTERNATIVES:

FATS:

TREATS AND SWEETS:

WATER:

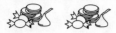

EXERCISE:

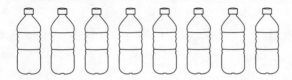

PORTION TELLER PROGRESS:

portion teller progress sheet

Record number of servings per day consumed from each food group along with any portion progress for the week.

FOOD GROUP	MON	TUES	WED	THURS	FRI	SAT	SUN
FRUITS: 2-4 servings daily							
VEGETABLES: 3 + servings daily							
GRAINS AND STARCHY VEGETABLES: 4-8 servings daily							
DAIRY: 2-3 servings daily							
FISH, POULTRY, MEATS, AND ALTERNATIVES: 2-3 servings daily							
FATS: 1-3 servings daily							
TREATS/SWEETS: 0-2 servings daily							
PORTION TELLER PROGRESS:							

serving sizes of most foods in all food groups

nonstarchy vegetables:

3+ servings daily

1 cup raw = 1 baseball
½ cup cooked = ½ baseball

Alfalfa sprouts

Artichokes

Asparagus

Bamboo shoots

Bean sprouts

Beets

Broccoli

Brussels sprouts

Cabbage

Carrots

Cauliflower

Celery

Cucumber

Eggplant

Fennel

Green beans

Greens (collards, kale, mustard, turnip)

Kohlrabi

Leeks

Mushrooms

Okra

Onions

Pea pods

Peppers (red, yellow, green)

Radishes

Salad greens (arugula, endive, escarole, assorted lettuce, romaine)

Scallions

Snow peas

Spaghetti squash

Spinach

Sugar snap peas

Summer squash (yellow or zucchini)

Tomatoes

Water chestnuts

Watercress

Salsa, ½ cup	*½ baseball*
Tomato sauce, tomato puree, ½ cup	*½ baseball*
Tomato juice, 1 cup (8 fl oz)	*1 baseball*
V8 juice, 1 cup (8 fl oz)	*1 baseball*
Vegetable soup, 1 cup (8 fl oz)	*1 baseball*

Smart Bets: *All veggies, especially a colorful assortment. Nutrition superstars include asparagus, broccoli, carrots, red peppers, and spinach.*

Limit: *There's no need to avoid any vegetables. They are ALL good for you.*

fruit:

2 to 4 servings daily

Apple, 1	1 baseball
Applesauce, unsweetened, 1 cup	1 baseball
Apricots, fresh, 4 whole	
Banana, 1	
Berries (blackberries, blueberries, raspberries, strawberries), 1 cup	1 baseball
Canned fruit, unsweetened, 1 cup	1 baseball
Cantaloupe melon, 1 cup	1 baseball
Cherries, fresh, 1 cup	1 baseball
Clementines, 2	
Dried fruit, ¼ cup	1 golf ball
(e.g., 9 dried apricots, 4–5 prunes, small box of raisins, 2 dried figs)	
Figs, fresh, 2	
Fruit juice: orange, grapefruit, cranberry, 6 fl. oz	6-oz yogurt container
Fruit salad (assortment of mixed fruits), 1 cup	1 baseball
Grapefruit, ½	
Grapes, 1 cup	1 baseball
Honeydew, 1 cup	1 baseball
Kiwi fruit, 2	
Mango, ½, or 1 cup	1 baseball
Nectarine, 1	1 baseball
Orange, 1	1 baseball
Papaya, ½, or 1 cup	1 baseball
Peach, 1	1 baseball
Pear, 1	1 lightbulb
Persimmon, ½, or 1 cup	1 baseball
Pineapple, fresh, 1 cup	1 baseball
Plums, 2	

Tangerines, 2
Watermelon, 1 cup   **1 baseball**

Smart Bets: *All fresh fruits. Nutrition superstars include blueberries, kiwi fruit, citrus, and melons.*

Limit: *fruit juices, dried fruits, canned fruits in syrups*

grains and starchy vegetables:

4 to 8 servings daily

Starchy Vegetables

Cassava (yucca), ½ cup cooked   **½ baseball**
Corn, 1 ear
Corn, ½ cup cooked   **½ baseball**
Green peas, ½ cup cooked   **½ baseball**
Legumes (beans, peas, and lentils),* ½ cup cooked   **½ baseball**
    Black-eyed peas, black beans, chick peas (garbanzo beans),
    kidney beans, lentils, lima beans, pinto beans, split peas, white beans
Parsnip, ½ cup cooked   **½ baseball**
Plantain, ½ cup cooked   **½ baseball**
Potato, baked with skin, ½, about 3–4 oz, or ½ cup   **½ computer mouse**
Potato, boiled, ½ cup   **½ baseball**
Pumpkin, ½ cup cooked   **½ baseball**
Rutabaga, ½ cup cooked   **½ baseball**
Sweet potato, yam, baked, ½, about 3–4 oz, or ½ cup **½ computer mouse**
Winter squash (butternut, acorn, pumpkin), 1 cup cooked   **1 baseball**

*NOTE: Legumes also can be counted as a meat alternative. Do not count in both groups.

Whole Grains or Healthy Grains

Amaranth, ½ cooked	½ *baseball*
Barley, ½ cup cooked	½ *baseball*
Bread slice, whole-grain (whole-wheat, rye, oat), 1 oz	1 *CD case*
Bulgur (tabouli), ½ cup cooked	½ *baseball*

Cereal:

Ready-to-eat (cold) unsweetened cereal, whole-grain, approximately 1 oz	
Puffed wheat or puffed brown rice, 2 cups	2 *baseballs*
Flakes (bran, corn, oat), 1 cup	1 *baseball*
Oat rings (Cheerios), 1 cup	1 *baseball*
Brown rice cereal, 1 cup	1 *baseball*
Shredded Wheat (1 biscuit)	
Spoon-size Shredded Wheat, ½ cup	½ *baseball*
Low-fat granola, nuggets, muesli, ¼ cup	1 *golf ball*

Cooked cereal:

Whole-grain, ⅔ cup cooked (⅓ cup uncooked or 1 packet)	1 *tennis ball*
Buckwheat groats, ⅔ cup cooked	1 *tennis ball*
Cracked wheat, ⅔ cup cooked	1 *tennis ball*
Oat bran, ⅔ cup cooked	1 *tennis ball*
Oatmeal, ⅔ cup cooked	1 *tennis ball*
Wheatena, ⅔ cup cooked	1 *tennis ball*

Cereal or granola bar, whole-grain, 1, 1 oz	
Couscous, whole-wheat, ½ cup cooked	½ *baseball*
Crackers, whole-grain varieties, 1 oz	*CD case*
2–3 large (size of whole-grain crisp bread such as Ryvita, Kavli, Finn Crisp)	
3 breadsticks, whole-wheat, approx 4½ in	
5–6 small (size of whole grain Wheat Thins)	
Kasha (buckwheat groats), ½ cup cooked	½ *baseball*
Matzo board, whole-wheat, 1	
Millet, ½ cup cooked	½ *baseball*

Pancake, whole-grain varieties, 1 (1 oz or about
4 inches across)   ***diameter of CD***
Pasta, whole-wheat, ½ cup cooked   ***½ baseball***
Pita, whole-wheat, 1 (1 oz or about 4 inches across)   ***diameter of CD***
    Pita, large, 2 oz = 2 servings
Popcorn, air-popped (microwave, no fat added), 3 cups   ***3 baseballs***
Pretzels, whole-wheat or oat-bran, 1 oz (¾ cup, small bag) ***1 tennis ball***
Quinoa, ½ cup cooked   ***½ baseball***
Rice, brown or wild, ½ cup cooked   ***½ baseball***
Rice cakes, 2 regular size (4 inches) or 10 mini   ***diameter of 2 CDs***
Soba noodles, ½ cup cooked   ***½ baseball***
Tortilla, whole-wheat, 1 ounce (7-inch)
    Large tortilla, 2 oz = 2 servings
Waffle, whole-grain varieties, 1 (1 oz or about
    4 inches square)   ***diameter of CD***
Wheat germ, 3 Tbsp   ***1½ walnuts***

White-Flour Products

Sliced white bread, pita, tortilla, waffles, pancakes, cereals (the same
serving sizes as for whole grains apply here)
Crackers: 1 oz   ***1 CD case***
    2–3 large crackers (size of graham crackers)
    2–3 breadsticks
    5–6 small crackers (size of saltines)
    8 animal crackers
    24 oyster crackers
Pasta (spaghetti, macaroni, lasagna noodles), ½ cup cooked ***½ baseball***
Pretzels, 1 oz (¾ cup)   ***1 tennis ball***
    1 Bavarian/Baldie
    2 pretzel rods
    9 three-ring, 20 mini-twists
    48 sticks
Rice, white, ½ cup cooked   ***½ baseball***
Taco shells, corn, 2 (6-inch)

Smart Bets: *whole-grain breads and cereals (whole-wheat, rye, oat), cooked cereal, such as oatmeal and Wheatena; brown rice, kasha, bulgur, barley; all starchy vegetables, such as sweet potatoes, corn, winter squash; legumes such as lentils, chick peas, and kidney beans*

Limit: *white-flour products, such as white bread, pasta, bagels, crackers, muffins, pretzels, white rice; cereals with added sugar; and, of course, beware of giant-size bread products*

Healthy Hints: *Pay special attention to single-serve items that are available in huge sizes: muffins, bagels, street pretzels, and knishes. Even if you're buying "brown" bread, you can't be sure it's made from the whole-wheat flour. Always read the label for the words "whole wheat" before buying "health" bread products.*

fish, poultry, meat, and meat alternatives:

2 to 3 servings daily

(approximately 6 to 8 ounces)

Fish, Poultry, Meat

3 oz cooked   **1 deck of cards**

   Beef

   Chicken

   Cornish hen

   Fish (bass, cod, flounder, haddock, halibut, grouper,
      ocean perch, red snapper, salmon, sardines, sole,
      swordfish, tuna)

   Game (buffalo, venison)

   Lamb

Liver
Pork
Seafood (shrimp, scallops, lobster, oysters)
Turkey
Veal

Meat Alternatives

Eggs, 2	
Egg substitute, ½ cup	
Egg whites, 4–6	
Hummus, ½ cup	*½ baseball*
Legumes (beans, peas, lentils), 1 cup cooked	*1 baseball*
Bean (split pea, white bean) or lentil soup, 1 cup	*1 baseball*
Soy/veggie burger, 1 (3 oz)	*1 deck of cards*
Textured vegetable protein, 3 oz	*1 deck of cards*
Tofu or tempeh, 1 cup	*1 baseball*

*NOTE: Protein in 1 oz meat/fish/poultry = 1 egg, 2 egg whites, ½ cup cooked legumes

Smart Bets: *Poultry (without skin), fish, and meat alternatives. Include leaner cuts of beef (USDA Select or Choice grades, trimmed, such as round, sirloin, and flank steak; tenderloin; roast; T-bone).*

Limit: *processed sandwich meats such as salami, bologna, sausage; hot dogs; bacon and spareribs*

Healthy Hints: *Try to eat a little bit of protein with each meal (with the emphasis on "little"). Don't pile all your meat for the entire day into one meal—spread it out during the day. Limit red meat to once or twice a week. And watch your portions! Don't exceed more than 2 servings of fish, poultry, or meat (6 ounces cooked) at one sitting. Try to have fish at least twice a week. Try to have one meat alternative daily.*

dairy: 2 to 3 servings daily

Fat-Free, Low-Fat, and Reduced-Fat Dairy

Buttermilk, fat-free or low-fat, 1 cup	*1 baseball*
Cheese, Parmesan, grated, 3–4 Tbsp	*1½–2 walnuts*
Cottage cheese, fat-free or low-fat, ½ cup	*½ baseball*
Evaporated fat-free milk, ½ cup	*½ baseball*
Farmer cheese, fat-free or low-fat, ¼ cup, or reduced-fat,	*1 golf ball*
Hard cheese, fat-free, part-skim, or low-fat, 2 slices,	*6–8 dice*
2 slices, 1½–2 oz (e.g., Jarlsberg, part-skim mozzarella, reduced-fat feta, reduced-fat Swiss, 2 rounds of Laughing Cow Light or Mini Babybell Light)	
Hoop cheese, ½ cup	*rounded handful*
Ice milk, 1 cup	*1 baseball*
Milk, fat-free or low-fat (1%), 1 cup or 8 fl oz	*1 baseball*
Pot cheese, ½ cup	*rounded handful*
Ricotta cheese, part-skim, ¼ cup	*1 golf ball*
Soy milk, calcium-fortified, fat-free or low-fat,	
1 cup (not technically a dairy, but a good dairy substitute)	*1 baseball*
Yogurt, fat-free or low-fat, 1 cup or 8 fl oz	*1 container*

Whole-Milk Dairy

Cheese, whole-milk varieties, 2 slices, 1½–2 oz	
(American, Brie, cheddar, Monterey Jack)	*6–8 dice*
Evaporated whole milk, ½ cup or 4 fl oz	*½ baseball*
Goat's milk, 1 cup or 8 fl oz	*1 baseball*
Kefir, 1 cup or 8 fl oz	*1 baseball*
Whole milk, 1 cup or 8 fl oz	*1 baseball*
Yogurt, whole milk, 1 cup or 8 fl oz	*1 container*

Smart Bets: *fat-free, low-fat, and part-skim dairy products*

Limit: *whole-milk dairy*

Healthful Hints: *Include some dairy for breakfast or an afternoon snack; it's a great source of protein. It's much better to eat your dairy than to pop a pill.*

fat: 1 to 3 servings daily

Healthy Fats

Avocado, ¼ medium	
Nuts (peanuts, cashews, almonds, walnuts, pistachios), 1 oz (about ¼ cup)	*1 golf ball*
Oil (canola, corn, olive, peanut, safflower, sesame, soybean), 1 Tbsp (3 tsp)	*½ shot glass*
Olives, 12–15 medium	
Peanut butter and other nut butters, 1 Tbsp	*½ walnut or 3 standard postal stamps*
Salad dressing (olive-oil based), 1 Tbsp	*½ shot glass*
Salad dressing, reduced fat, 2 Tbsp	*shot glass*
Seeds (sesame, sunflower, pumpkin), 1 oz (about ¼ cup)	*golf ball*
Tahini paste, 1 Tbsp	*½ walnut*

Unhealthy Fats

Butter, 1 Tbsp	*½ walnut or 3 standard postal stamps*
Coconut, shredded, 3 Tbsp	*1½ walnuts*
Cream, half-and-half, 2 Tbsp	*1 walnut*
Cream cheese, 1 Tbsp	*½ walnut*
Margarine, 1 Tbsp	*½ walnut*

Mayonnaise, 1 Tbsp	*½ walnut*
Salad dressing (creamy), 1 Tbsp	*½ shot glass*
Sour cream, 3 Tbsp	*1½ walnuts*

Smart Bets: *healthy fats such as olive oil, canola oil, most vegetable oils, tahini, avocado, olives, nuts, nut butters, and seeds*

Limit: *unhealthy fats such as butter, coconut oil, cream cheese, margarine, mayonnaise, and creamy salad dressing*

treats and sweets:

0–2 servings daily

Alcoholic beverages	
5–6 fl oz wine	*6-oz yogurt container*
12 fl oz beer	*12-fl-oz can*
Cakes and cookies, 1 oz	
Biscotti, 1	
Cookies, 2 (2-in)	*2 tea bags or 2 Oreo cookies*
Cake sliver, 1 oz	*CD case*
Cupcake, mini, 1 oz	*half-dollar size across*
Gingersnaps, 2 (2-in)	*2 tea bags or 2 Oreo cookies*
Pie, ⅓ cup	*golf ball, 4–5 forkfuls*
Candies and sweets, ¼ cup unless	
indicated	*1 golf ball or 1 layer on your palm*
Chocolate	
1 mini, trick-or-treat-size bar	
2 small York Peppermint patties	
4 Hershey's Kisses	
M&M candies	*1 layer on your palm*

Cracker Jack, ½ cup   *½ baseball or 1 handful*
Fruit roll-up, 1
Gummy bears   *1 layer on your palm*
Hard candy, 3
Jelly beans   *1 layer on your palm*
Licorice, 2 twists
Lollipop, 1 Tootsie Pop or Charms Blow Pop
Tootsie Rolls, 3 midgies

Chips, ½ cup
  (e.g., 15 corn chips, 10 potato chips,
  15 soy crisps, 10 tortilla chips)   *1 handful or ½ baseball*

Energy/sports bar, 1 ounce   *1 Pria bar, ½ Balance bar, ½ Luna bar*

Fried foods
  French fries, ½ cup   *1 handful or ½ baseball*

Frozen treats
  Frozen fruit pop (frozen fruit), 1
  Fudgsicle pop, 1
  Ice cream, ½ cup   *½ baseball*
  Italian ice, ½ cup   *½ baseball*
  Frozen yogurt, ½ cup   *½ baseball*
  Low-fat or nonfat ice cream, ½ cup *½ baseball*
  Sorbet, ½ cup   *½ baseball*

Gravies and sauces, 2 Tbsp   *1 walnut in a shell*

Soft drinks, sugar-sweetened beverages, 8 oz   *small Styrofoam cup or 8-oz yogurt container*

Sugar, honey, jelly, maple syrup, 2 Tbsp   *walnut in a shell*

Lesser Evils:

Baked potato and tortilla chips: Baked Lays potato chips, Baked Doritos
Barry's French Twists
Fortune cookie
Frozen fruit pop (noncreamy varieties such as strawberry, raspberry, lemon, lime)
Jell-O

Low-fat or nonfat frozen yogurt or dietary dessert (TCBY, Tasti-D-Lite, Colombo)
Popsicle
"The Skinny Cow" Silhouette fudge bar or flying saucer, or ice cream sundae
Soy Crisps
Sorbet (noncreamy varieties such as mixed berry, raspberry, lemon)

water: 64 ounces water

8 (8-ounce) glasses daily:

water, seltzer, herbal tea

exercise: 30 minutes

3 to 4 times per week

the portion teller meal plans

BREAKFAST

For all breakfasts: you can include coffee or tea with fat-free or low-fat milk.

---

1 cup (8 oz) fat-free or low-fat yogurt, flavored or plain	*1 8-oz yogurt container*
1 cup fresh strawberries or blueberries	*1 baseball of berries*
Cereal for crunch (¼ cup low-fat granola, or Grape-Nuts) OR 1 muffin top (2 oz)	*1 golf ball of granola or cereal*

---

1 cup whole-grain, bran, oat, or other dry cereal (Multigrain Cheerios, Barbara's Cinnamon Puffins, Kashi Go Lean, bran flakes, Raisin Bran, etc.)	*1 baseball of cereal*

1 cup (8-oz) fat-free milk or 1% milk	*1 baseball of milk*
1 cup cantaloupe or melon in season	*1 baseball of cantaloupe or melon*

½ pink grapefruit OR 1 orange or ¾ cup (6 fl oz) fresh squeezed citrus juice	*6-oz yogurt container of juice*
3–4 egg whites, omelet or scrambled	
Assorted vegetables—tomatoes, spinach, mushrooms	*1 handful of veggies*
1 slice part-skim cheese, optional	*1 CD of cheese*
1 slice whole-grain toast or 2–3 whole-grain crackers (Kavli or Ryvitas)	*1 CD case of toast or crackers*
1 Tbsp fruit jam, optional	*½ walnut shell of jam*

1-oz pita (whole-wheat preferred)	*1 pita the diameter of a CD*
1 slice melted part-skim cheese	*1 CD of cheese*
2–3 slices tomato, optional	
1 cup fruit salad (melon, berries, sliced apple)	*1 tight fist of fruit salad*

---

1 toasted English muffin (whole-wheat, oat-bran preferred)

¼ cup farmer cheese or part-skim ricotta sprinkled with cinnamon and nutmeg	*1 golf ball of cheese*
1 Tbsp chopped walnuts, optional	*½ walnut shell of chopped nuts*
1 cup fresh pineapple or fruit of choice	*1 baseball of fruit*

½ bagel or 1 English muffin (whole-wheat or oat-bran preferred)

1 Tbsp low-fat cream cheese	*½ walnut shell of cream cheese*
2 slices lox or smoked salmon	*2 matchbooks of smoked salmon*
2–3 slices fresh tomato	
1 orange or 6 fl oz orange juice	*1 baseball-sized orange or 6-oz yogurt container of juice*

---

2 cups Puffed Wheat cereal	*2 baseballs of cereal*
1 glass (8-oz) nonfat or low-fat milk	*1 yogurt container of milk*
1 cup mixed berries	*1 baseball of berries*

---

1 whole-grain waffle or pancake (about 4 inches in diameter)	*1 waffle or pancake the diameter of a CD*
1 cup fresh banana	*1 baseball of bananas*
1 Tbsp peanut butter	*½ walnut of peanut butter*
4 oz yogurt or milk, fat-free or low-fat	*½ baseball of yogurt or milk*

Fruit Smoothie:

½ cup fat-free milk	*½ baseball of milk*
½ cup plain or vanilla yogurt	*½ baseball of yogurt*
½ banana	
½ cup strawberries	*½ baseball of strawberries*
½ cup orange juice	*½ baseball of juice*
Ice	

½ cantaloupe	*2 baseballs of cantaloupe*
½ cup low-fat or fat-free cottage cheese	*½ baseball of cottage cheese*
¼ cup low-fat granola or crunchy cereal, or 1 slice raisin toast	*1 golf ball of cereal* *1 CD case of toast*

1 slice whole-grain toast	**1 CD case of toast**
1 scrambled or poached egg	
¼ cup (1 oz) part-skim mozzarella cheese, optional	**4 dice of cheese**
2 kiwi fruit or 1 cup strawberries	**1 baseball of kiwi or strawberries**

⅔ cup cooked oatmeal (1 packet or ⅓ cup dry)	**1 tennis ball of oatmeal**
6 oz fat-free milk or vanilla soymilk	**6-oz yogurt container**
1 cup mixed berries dash of cinnamon, vanilla, and 1 tsp of sugar, optional	**1 baseball of berries**

LUNCH

1 cup of vegetable or minestrone soup, 8 oz

1 baseball of soup

Pita pocket sandwich:

3-oz fresh turkey, grilled chicken, grilled salmon, OR ½ cup hummus

1 deck of cards of poultry or fish, or ½ baseball of hummus

1 whole-wheat pita (1 oz, 4 inches across)

1 pita the diameter of a CD

Lettuce, tomato, and shredded carrots

1 handful of veggies

1–2 tsp salad dressing

1–2 water bottle capfuls of dressing

Mustard or ketchup, optional

Grilled chicken breast (or grilled salmon) salad platter:

3 oz grilled chicken breast (or salmon)

1 deck of cards of meat

Large tossed salad with your favorite fresh vegetables

2 baseballs of salad

1 Tbsp salad dressing or olive oil, unlimited balsamic vinegar, fresh lemon, and spices to taste

½ shot glass of dressing, or oil

4–5 egg-white omelet with spinach and/or broccoli, mushrooms, and tomatoes	*1 handful of veggies*
2 slices part-skim cheese, 2 oz	*2 CDs of cheese*
Salad of romaine lettuce, sliced tomato, and cucumber	*2 baseballs of salad*
1 Tbsp salad dressing or olive oil, unlimited balsamic vinegar, fresh lemon, and spices to taste	*½ shot glass of dressing, or oil*
1 slice whole-wheat or rye toast with 1 tsp butter	*1 CD case of toast* *1 thumptip of butter*

Tuna melt:

3 oz water-packed tuna	*1 deck of cards of tuna*
Honey mustard	
1 Tbsp mayonnaise	*½ walnut shell of mayonnaise*
Shredded carrots, chopped celery	*1 tennis ball of carrots and celery*
English muffin (whole-wheat or oat-bran preferred) OR 2 slices whole-wheat toast	*2 CD cases*
Sliced tomato	
1 oz part-skim cheese	*4 dice of cheese*

Large chopped salad with vegetables of choice:

Unlimited lettuce, cucumber, tomato,
peppers, carrots, and veggies of choice

1 Tbsp salad dressing or olive oil, unlimited
balsamic vinegar, fresh lemon, and spices
to taste

½ shot glass of dressing, or oil

1 hard-boiled egg or ½ cup tofu

½ baseball tofu

½ cup chick peas or black beans

½ baseball of chick peas or black beans

½ cup corn

½ baseball of corn

1 to 2 whole-grain bread sticks, optional

Turkey wrap:

1 flour tortilla (whole-wheat preferred, 1 oz,
6 inches across)

1½ CDs of tortilla

2 Tbsps cranberry sauce

1 walnut shell of cranberry sauce

3 oz fresh turkey breast

1 deck of cards of turkey

½ thinly sliced apple

½ tennis ball of apple

A few lettuce leaves

½ baseball of lettuce

1 slice vegetable pizza, topped with spinach, tomato, broccoli, or vegetable of choice	*2–3 CD cases of bread* *2 CDs of cheese* *1 baseball of veggies* *and sauce*
Chopped lettuce, tomato, and cucumber salad	*2 baseballs of salad*
1 Tbsp salad dressing or olive oil, unlimited balsamic vinegar, fresh lemon, and spices to taste	*½ shot glass of dressing,* *or oil*
1 tsp Parmesan cheese, pepper, and oregano	*1 standard postal stamp* *of Parmesan cheese*

Fresh fruit platter:

2 cups fruit salad of strawberries, assorted melons, and kiwi OR ½ cantaloupe	*2 baseballs of fruit*
½ cup low-fat cottage cheese or pot cheese sprinkled with cinnamon OR 1 cup low-fat yogurt	*½ baseball cheese* *OR 1 (8 oz) yogurt* *container*
2 slices raisin toast OR ½ small bran muffin	*2 CD cases of toast OR* *½ tennis ball of bran* *muffin*

Stuffed baked potato:

1 baked potato (7 oz)   *1 computer mouse-sized potato*

Steamed broccoli, spinach, OR vegetables of   *1 baseball of veggies*
choice

¼ cup part-skim shredded cheese OR 1 cup   *1 golf ball of cheese OR*
vegetarian chili OR yogurt   *1 baseball of chili or*
                                                            yogurt

Fresh spinach and mushroom salad topped with grilled chicken:

2 cups fresh spinach and mushrooms   *2 baseballs of salad*

Grilled chicken breast, 3 oz   *1 deck of cards of chicken*

2 Tbsps low-fat raspberry vinaigrette dressing   *1 shot glass of dressing*

2 Tbsps slivered almonds   *1 shot glass of almonds*

3 Kavli Crispsbread, Finn Crisps, or Ryvita
(optional)

1 veggie burger OR turkey burger

Whole-wheat pita (1 oz)   *1 pita the diameter
                                                         of a CD*

Lettuce, tomato, and shredded carrots   *½ baseball of veggies*

Mustard or ketchup, optional

Tossed salad   *1 baseball of salad*

1 Tbsp salad dressing or olive oil, unlimited   *½ shot glass of dressing,
balsamic vinegar, fresh lemon, and spices   or oil*
to taste

Homemade pita pizza:

2 oz pita (whole-wheat preferred)   *1 pita the diameter of
                                                    approximately 2 CDs*

½ cup marinara sauce OR fresh tomato sauce   *½ baseball of sauce*

¼ cup part-skim mozzarella cheese   *1 golf ball of cheese*

Mushrooms, tomatoes, onions, and peppers   *1 tennis ball of veggies*

DINNER

Bowl of vegetable or minestrone soup, 12 oz, OR garden salad of romaine lettuce, tomato, mushrooms, and peppers with 1 Tbsp salad dressing or olive oil, unlimited balsamic vinegar, fresh lemon, and spices to taste	*1½ 8-oz yogurt containers of soup OR 2 baseballs of salad with ½ shot glass of dressing, or oil*
3–4 ounces grilled OR broiled salmon OR tuna OR sea bass	*1 deck of cards of fish*
Grilled vegetables with 1–2 tsp olive oil OR steamed vegetables with salsa OR tomato sauce	*1 baseball of veggies with 1–2 caps of a water bottle of oil OR 1 baseball of veggies with ½ baseball of salsa or sauce*
½ cup rice pilaf, kasha, OR tabouli	*½ baseball of grain*

Large salad with endive, radicchio, peppers, and cherry tomatoes	*2 baseballs of salad*
1 Tbsp salad dressing or olive oil, unlimited balsamic vinegar, fresh lemon, and spices to taste	*½ shot glass of dressing, or oil*
3–4 oz baked OR broiled chicken breast OR sirloin steak	*1 deck of cards of chicken or steak*

1 cup broccoli OR fresh asparagus sautéed in olive oil	*1 baseball of veggies*
1 sweet potato (6 oz) OR 1 baked potato (6 oz) topped with fresh tomato sauce OR 1 cup butternut squash	*1computer mouse–sized potato with ½ baseball of sauce OR 1 baseball of squash*

Mixed green salad	*2 tight fists of salad*
1 Tbsp salad dressing or olive oil, unlimited balsamic vinegar, fresh lemon, and spices to taste	*½ shot glass of dressing, or oil*

Pasta primavera:

1½ cups pasta (whole-wheat preferred)	*1½ baseballs of pasta*
Steamed mixed vegetables as desired: cauliflower, broccoli, carrots, eggplant, peppers	*1 baseball of mixed veggies*
Fresh tomato OR marinara sauce	*½ baseball of sauce*
3 Tbsp Parmesan cheese, optional	*1½ walnut shells of cheese*

NOTE: This meal can be ordered at your local Italian restaurant.

Chopped salad:

Tomato and cucumber salad	*2 baseballs of salad*
Feta cheese, 1 oz	*4 dice*
1 Tbsp salad dressing or olive oil, unlimited balsamic vinegar, fresh lemon, and spices to taste	*½ shot glass of dressing, or oil*
3–4 oz flounder, filet of sole, OR red snapper broiled or baked with lemon, parsley, a drizzle of oil and spices OR 1 cup lentils, chick peas OR your favorite bean dish	*1 checkbook of fish OR 1 baseball of beans*
Steamed vegetables with 1 tsp olive oil, fresh garlic, lemon and spices OR 1 cup spaghetti squash topped with fresh tomatoes	*1 baseball of veggies with 1–2 caps of a water bottle of oil OR 1 baseball of spaghetti squash*
1 cup couscous, brown rice, OR barley	*1 baseball of grain*

Miso soup OR small green salad with 1 Tbsp carrot ginger dressing	*1 baseball or 8-oz yogurt container of soup or salad with ½ walnut shell of dressing*
Chicken (OR salmon) teriyaki: 4–5 oz chicken (OR salmon)	*1½ deck of cards of chicken or fish*
Assorted vegetables of choice (1 cup cooked)	*1 baseball of veggies*
Teriyaki sauce	
1 cup cooked brown rice	*1 baseball of rice*

NOTE: This meal can be ordered at your local Japanese restaurant.

1 cup vegetable or chicken broth	*1 baseball or 8-oz yogurt container of broth*
Large platter of mixed steamed vegetables	*2 baseballs of mixed veggies*
1 cup brown rice OR 4 steamed vegetable dumplings	*1 baseball of rice*
1 cup tofu OR 3 oz chicken	*1 baseball of tofu OR 1 deck of cards of chicken*
Ginger sauce, garlic sauce, OR your favorite sauce, 1 Tbsp	*½ walnut shell of sauce*

NOTE: This meal can be ordered at your local Chinese restaurant.

Tossed garden salad of romaine lettuce, tomato, mushrooms, and vegetables of choice	*2 baseballs of salad*
1 Tbsp salad dressing or olive oil, unlimited balsamic vinegar, fresh lemon, and spices to taste	*½ shot glass of dressing, or oil*
3–4 oz roast turkey breast	*Palm of your hand of turkey*
¼ cup cranberry sauce	*1 golf ball of sauce*
2 Tbsps gravy, optional	*1 walnut shell of gravy*
1 cup mixed vegetables sautéed in 1 tsp olive oil	*1 baseball of veggies in 1 thumb tip of oil*
1 baked sweet potato (6 oz) OR 1 cup acorn squash topped with a dash of cinnamon and nutmeg	*1 sweet potato the size of a computer mouse or a baseball of acorn squash*

Chopped tomato and cucumber salad	*2 baseballs of salad*
1 Tbsp salad dressing or olive oil, unlimited balsamic vinegar, fresh lemon, and spices to taste	*½ shot glass of dressing, or oil*
Baked chicken breast (6 oz) brushed with barbeque sauce, 2 Tbsps	*2 decks of cards of chicken 1 shot glass*
1 ear of corn on the cob with 1–2 tsp trans-fat-free margarine OR butter, or ½ cup wild rice	*1–2 thumb tips of margarine OR butter, OR ½ baseball of rice*

2 cups steamed mixed vegetables	*2 baseballs of mixed veggies*

Salad with endive, radicchio, peppers, and cherry tomatoes	*2 tight fists of salad*
1 Tbsp salad dressing or olive oil, unlimited balsamic vinegar, fresh lemon, and spices to taste	*½ shot glass of dressing, or oil*

Spaghetti squash primavera:

2–3 cups spaghetti squash, baked eggplant, and zucchini	*2–3 baseballs of veggies*
1 cup fresh tomato sauce	*1 baseball of sauce*
3 Tbsps Parmesan cheese	*1½ walnut shells of cheese*

Tossed salad with dressing	*2 baseballs salad with ½ walnut shell of dressing*

Spinach and feta cheese omelet:
    2 eggs OR 4 egg whites

2 oz feta cheese	*8 dice of cheese*
chopped spinach	*1 baseball of spinach*

Baked potato with 1–2 tsp butter or 2 slices whole-wheat toast with 1–2 tsp butter	*1 computer mouse–sized potato with 1–2 thumb tips butter or 2 CD cases of toast with 1–2 thumb tips of butter*

NOTE: This meal can be ordered at your local diner.

Mixed salad with fresh vegetables of choice	*2 baseballs salad*
1 Tbsp salad dressing or olive oil, unlimited balsamic vinegar, fresh lemon, and spices to taste	*½ shot glass of dressing, or oil*
3–4 oz broiled sirloin steak or salmon steak	*1 deck of cards steak or salmon*
1 cup broccoli, cauliflower, and carrots sauteed in 1 tsp oil	*1 baseball veggies, 1 thumb tip oil*
½ cup brown rice or couscous	*½ baseball*

Green salad with 1 Tbsp carrot ginger dressing OR seaweed salad	*2 handfuls of salad with ½ walnut shell of dressing*
Edamame (steamed soy beans)—share a side order	*½ baseball of edamame*
2 (6-pieces) rolls sushi (tuna, salmon, yellowtail, California Roll, etc.)	
Oshitashi (steamed spinach)	*1 baseball of spinach*

NOTE: This meal can be ordered at your local Japanese restaurant.

SNACKS

1 cup fresh mixed berries (blueberries, raspberries, and strawberries)	*1 baseball of berries*
Fresh fruit salad of watermelon, cantaloupe, kiwi, etc., 2 cups, topped with 1 Tbsp wheat germ, optional	*2 baseballs of fruit salad with ½ walnut shell of wheat germ*
1 cup low-fat vanilla frozen yogurt OR ice cream (soft serve)—small order	*1 8-oz yogurt container of frozen yogurt OR ice cream*

Fresh fruit shake:

1 cup bananas, strawberries, kiwi	**1 baseball of fruit**
4-oz skim milk, ice as desired	**½ baseball of skim milk**

1–2 cups baby carrots and celery sticks with salsa or hummus, 1 Tbsp	**1–2 baseballs of veggies with 1 golf ball salsa or hummus**

1 apple OR 1 cup unsweetened apple sauce OR 1 baked apple	**1 baseball-sized apple OR of applesauce**

Raspberry or strawberry frozen fruit pop OR sorbet pop

Chocolate shake: 1 glass skim milk	**1 yogurt container of milk**
1 Tbsp chocolate syrup, ice as desired	**½ walnut shell of syrup**

3 cups air popped popcorn (sprinkled with 1 Tbsp Parmesan cheese, optional)	**6 handfuls of popcorn ½ walnut shell**

Frozen banana: peel and sprinkle with cinnamon or chocolate syrup or a schmear of peanut butter before freezing	**½ walnut shell of peanut butter**

1 cup grapes or frozen grapes	**1 tight fist of grapes**

Small bag pretzels, 1 oz	*1 tennis ball of pretzels*
1 multi-grain cereal bar or low-fat granola bar	
1 Pria bar or ½ Balance bar	
1 cup low-fat yogurt topped with ¼ cup of mixed nuts and raisins	*1 (8-oz) yogurt container* *1 golf ball of nuts and raisins*
2 graham crackers (or an apple) and 1 Tbsp peanut butter or almond butter	*1 baseball-sized apple and ½ walnut shell of peanut or almond butter*
Small bag of soy chips or Baked Lays and a cup of V8 or tomato juice	*1–1.5-oz bag of chips and (8-oz) yogurt container of juice*
1 fudge pop OR ice cream sandwich OR flying saucer (Skinny Cow)	

· appendix f ·

size-inflation time line

Landmark Dates in the Supersizing of the American Candy Bar

1908   *The first Hershey Milk Chocolate Bar weighs 0.6 ounce.*

1960   *The Hershey Milk Chocolate Bar now weighs 1 ounce.*

1970   *M&M/Mars introduces the King-size Snickers.*

1976   *The Hershey Milk Chocolate Bar goes up to 1.4 ounce.*

1979   *Hershey Foods gets rid of the 8-ounce and 16-ounce cans of Hershey's Chocolate Syrup, replacing them with the 24-ounce bottle.*

1980   *Hershey Foods introduces the Big Block, a 2.6-ounce bar for its popular Milk Chocolate, Almond, and Krackle varieties.*

   •   *M&M/Mars increases the size of Snickers, M&Ms, Three Musketeers, and other chocolate candy bars, but keeps the price the same.*

1981   *M&M/Mars introduces the King-size M&Ms.*

   •   *The Hershey's Milk Chocolate Bar now weighs 1.5 ounces.*

1982   *M&M/Mars increases the size of chocolate candy bars yet again!*

1984   *Movie-theater chocolate candy bars now weigh 25% more; for example, the Nestlé Crunch is 3.5 ounces.*

1986   *Chocolate candy bars continue to grow—Hershey Foods increases the Milk Chocolate Bar to 1.7 ounces.*

1987   *Hershey Foods introduces King-size Reese's Peanut Butter Cup.*

1988   *Hershey Foods introduces the King-size Kit Kat.*

   •   *Theater candy bars continue to grow. The Kit Kat bar is double its original weight.*

1989   *M&M/Mars introduces the King-size Milky Way.*

1991   *The Hershey Big Block bars are renamed King-size.*

1992   *M&M/Mars introduces King-size Twix.*

   •   *Nestlé's bars multiply in size with the introduction of the King-size bar, at almost twice the size of a Regular bar, and the Giant-size, at three times the regular size.*

   •   *Nestlé offers three sizes of Nestlé Crunch bars: 1.6-ounce Regular, 2.8-ounce King, and 5-ounce Giant.*

   •   *Nestlé markets the Butterfinger Beast, a 5-ounce bar with nearly 700 calories.*

1997   *Goldenberg's jumps on the "more for less" bandwagon, increasing the King-size Peanut Chews from 2.7 ounces to 3.3 ounces, and advertising its regular bar with a slogan that says: "get 16% more free."*

1998   *M&M/Mars offers The Big One, a 3.7-ounce Snickers bar, 76% bigger than the regular-size bar.*

   •   *Hershey Foods advertises its Milk Chocolate Bar with the tag line: "14% free—get an 8-ounce bar at the 7-ounce price."*

2000   *Hershey Foods introduces the Big Kat, a full 27% bigger than the regular Kit Kat.*

2001   *Hershey Foods increases the King-size Kit Kat to 3 ounces, making it 100% larger than the regular Kit Kat.*

2003   *Nestlé promotes a 1.8-ounce Crunch bar with the label slogan: "10% more than the 1.6-ounce bar."*

   •   *Hershey Foods introduces the Reese's Peanut Butter Big Cup, one large 1.5-ounce cup.*

   •   *Hershey Foods offers a line of convenient single-serve bags of chocolate called ToGo for a variety of chocolates such as Mini Kisses, Kit Kat, and Reese's Bites, each weighing 2.8 ounces.*

   •   *Hershey Foods markets 12-ounce bags of individual snack-sized chocolates* that weigh 0.6 ounce each, which just happen to be the exact same size as the original chocolate bar introduced in 1908.

2004   The Hershey Milk Chocolate Bar is now available in these sizes: 1.6 ounces, 2.6 ounces, 4 ounces, 7 ounces, and 8 ounces. Quite a difference from the original 0.6 ounce bar! The smallest bar is more than 3 times the original size. And the largest bar is more than 13 times the original size!

Landmark Dates in the Supersizing of American Take-Out French Fries

1954   Burger King sells only Regular-size French fries, which weighs 2.6 ounces.

1955   McDonald's sells one size of French fries, called Fries, which weighs 2.4 ounces.

1972   McDonald's adds Large fries to the menu, weighing 3.5 ounces.

1985   McDonald's "Large fries for Small fries" promotion raises more than $2.6 million for Muscular Dystrophy.

1985   McDonald's increases the size of Large fries to 4.5 ounces. The former Large is now called Medium.

1988   McDonald's makes food history with Super-Size fries.

1989   Wendy's introduces the Super Value Menu which includes Biggie fries, weighing 5.6 ounces.

1991   Burger King offers Medium fries at 4.1 ounces.

1995   McDonald's discontinues Medium fries, offering Small, Large, and Super-Size.

•   McDonald's Large fries increases yet again to 5.3 ounces.

1997   Wendy's adds Great Biggie fries, at 6.7 ounces.

1999   Burger King offers Small (2.6 ounces), Medium (4.1 ounces), and King (6.1 ounces) fries.

•   McDonald's increases the weight of Super-Size fries by nearly one ounce, from 6.3 to 7.1 ounces. The former Super-Size is downgraded to a Large, and the Large becomes a Medium.

2001   Even though the Burger King Large was phased out in 1998, in favor of the

King, the company decides to make the King bigger by nearly an ounce (at 6.9 ounces), and add the Large size, weighing in at 5.7 ounces.

2002   Burger King discontinues Small fries in many locations. The Medium (4.1 ounces) is the smallest size available.

2003   McDonald's offers four sizes of fries: Small (2.4 ounces), Medium (5.3 ounces), Large (6.3 ounces), and Super-Size (7.1 ounces).

2004   McDonald's announces plan to discontinue the Super-Size except in special promotions. The largest size is the 6.3-ounce Large, the exact same weight as the 1998 Super-Size. Does it really make a difference if it is called Large or Super-Size? A huge order of fries is excessive no matter what it's called.

Landmark Dates in the Supersizing of the American Hamburger

1954   The first Burger King hamburger weighs 3.9 ounces, including the burger, bun, and toppings.

1955   The first McDonald's hamburger is 3.7 ounces, and contains 1.6 ounces of precooked beef.

1957   Burger King introduces the Whopper, with 4 ounces of precooked beef.

1968   Burger King has a new ad slogan: "The Bigger the Burger the Better the Burger."

   •   The Big Mac arrives at McDonald's, weighing 7.7 ounces and containing 3.2 ounces of precooked beef (twice as big as their original burger) with the tagline: "It's as good as it is big." (By today's standards, it would be small!)

1972   McDonald's adds the Quarter Pounder, containing 4 ounces of precooked beef, to the menu.

1982   Burger King competes with its fast-food competitors with the Bacon Double Cheeseburger.

1984   Wendy's introduces its famous "Where's the Beef?" advertising campaign to refute public perception that its burger is smaller than its competitors' "big name" burgers. The campaign is voted most popular commercial of 1984 and wins several advertising industry awards.

1986   Wendy's introduces the Big Bacon Classic, a quarter-pound beef patty topped with three slices of bacon, a slice of cheese, and a dollop of mayonnaise.

1988   Wendy's becomes the No. 3 bestselling fast-food chain by serving large burgers.

1993   McDonald's features the Mega Mac—two quarter-pound beef patties—five times bigger than its original burger.

1994   Burger King launches "Get Your Burger's Worth" campaign, increasing hamburgers (and other menu items like fries), by more than 50%.

1996   Sizzler advertises its new Bigger, Better Burger.

1997   McDonald's launches its popular "Just Super-Size Me" ad campaign: "For just 39 cents more, you get 20% more fries and 50% more drinks."

- McDonald's begins testing the Big Xtra (MBX), a 4.5-ounce patty advertised as containing 20% more beef than Burger King's Whopper.

- Jack in the Box introduces its Ultimate Burger.

- Burger King takes a hit at McDonald's with the Big King sandwich, advertised as "75% more beef than McDonald's Big Mac."

- Hardee's launches its Monster Burger.

1999   Burger King begins test marketing the half-pound Great American Burger.

2002   Jack in the Box beefs up the size of its burgers by 66% without raising its prices. It also begins using the larger patty for Jack's Kids Meals for an extra 10 cents.

- Wendy's markets the Classic Triple with Everything, including 3 slices of cheese, which weighs 14.5 ounces and has 1,030 calories.

- Burger King introduces the Meaty-Cheesy-Bacony X-Treme Whopper.

2003   Hardee's introduces Thickburgers, a line of hefty sandwiches where you get to choose by weight: a third-pound, a half-pound, or two-thirds of a pound. For low-carb lovers, you can now order the bunless version wrapped in lettuce.

- At Burger King, you can now choose five sizes of burgers, toppings and all: the 4.4-ounce Hamburger, the 6-ounce Whopper Jr., the 6.1-ounce Double Hamburger, the 9.9-ounce Whopper, and the 12.6-ounce Double Whopper (with nearly 1,000 calories). We've come a long way from the 3.9-ounce burger that BK opened with!

2004   Burger King offers a Triple cheeseburger.

- Carl's Jr. unveils its "double $6 burger" containing an entire pound of beef, three times the meat recommended for an average adult over an entire day.

- Hardee's introduces the Monster Thickburger—two ⅓-pound slabs of Angus beef, four strips of bacon, three slices of cheese and mayonnaise on a buttered sesame seed bun—packing 1,420 calories and 107 grams of fat. Add fries and a soda, and this single meal would involve more calories and fat than most people should get in an entire day.

Landmark Dates in the Supersizing of the American Pizza Pie

1975   Pizza Hut offers one pizza pie, 10 inches in diameter.

        Pizza Hut introduces a bigger pie, the Thick 'N Chewy pizza.

1979   Pizza Hut adds a 13-inch pie to the menu.

1983   Pizza Hut figures out how to pack more pie into a serving with the Personal Pan Pizza, an individual pizza pie that's bigger than a slice of pizza.

1984   Pizza Hut Big ups the size of their individual pizzas with the Topper pizza, a third larger than Personal Pan Pizza with 50% more cheese, that's meant to be eaten by one person in one sitting.

1992   Little Caesars introduces Pizza-by-the-Foot—you can now order a pizza as long as you are tall!

1993   Pizza Hut introduces the BIGFOOT Pizza, two square feet of pizza.

        Domino's introduces the Dominator Pizza, a 10- by 30-inch rectangle.

1995   Pizza Hut makes more of the crust with Stuffed Crust Pizza, 14 inches in diameter.

1996   Pizza Hut does it again with the TripleDecker Pizza, featuring a six-cheese blend sealed between two layers of crust.

1997   Little Caesars makes all of its pizzas bigger, increasing small pizzas from 10 to 14 inches, medium from 12 to 16 inches, and large from 16 to 18 inches, and adds the BIG! BIG! Pizza to the menu, along with the press release, "Bigger is better!"

1998   California Pizza Kitchen phases out the 9-inch pizza in favor of 10 inches.

2000   Pizza Hut introduces The Big New Yorker Pizza, a "bigger 16-inch crust with large, holdable, foldable slices."

2002   Pizza Hut makes a 12-inch Medium, a 14-inch Large, and a 16-inch Big New Yorker. Anyone want a Small? Too bad—it's not on the menu, unless you want the Personal Pan at 6 inches.

2004   Domino's introduces the Doublemelt pizza

- Pizza Hut unveils the Full House XL Pizza, touted as being 30% bigger than its regular pizza.

Landmark Dates in the Supersizing of the American Take-Out Soft Drinks

1954   Burger King offers a 12-ounce Small and a 16-ounce Large soft drink.

1955   McDonald's offers a 7-ounce soft drink.

1961   McDonald's adds the 12-ounce drink.

1962   McDonald's adds the 16-ounce drink.

1973   7-Eleven introduces 12- and 20-ounce-soda sizes.

1974   McDonald's adds the 21-ounce drink.

1976   7-Eleven starts an upward trend with the 16-ounce Gulp.

1978   7-Eleven adds the 32-ounce Big Gulp.

1983   7-Eleven adds the 44-ounce Super Big Gulp.

1988   McDonald's jumps on the big bandwagon with the 32-ounce Super-Size drink, a quart of soda.

- 7-Eleven tops them all with the 64-ounce Double Gulp drink—a half gallon of soda with nearly 800 calories!

1989   Wendy's adds the Super Value Menu that includes Biggie drinks.

1999   McDonald's introduces the 42-ounce Super-Size drink. The 32-ounce Super-Size is downgraded to simply Large.

2001   Burger King introduces a 42-ounce King drink.

2003   7-Eleven gets rid of the 16-ounce size, replacing it with the 20-ounce Gulp.

You can choose these drink sizes at 7-Eleven: 20-ounce, 32-ounce, 44-ounce, and 64-ounce.

At McDonald's, you can choose these drink sizes: 12-ounce Child, 16-ounce Small, 21-ounce Medium, 32-ounce Large, and 42-ounce Super-Size.

At Burger King, you can choose these drink sizes: 12-ounce Kiddie, 16-ounce Small, 22-ounce Medium, 32-ounce Large, and 42-ounce King.

2004   *McDonald's announces plans to phase out the 42-ounce Super-Size, except in special promotions. The largest size is the 32-ounce Large: a quart of soda, marketed for one person.*

• references •

American Dietetic Association. *Nutrition and You: Trends 2002. ADA Survey Shows Americans Can Use Some Help in Sizing Up Their Meals,* http://www.eatright.org.

American Institute for Cancer Research. "Amid Obesity Epidemic, More Americans Than Ever Are Cleaning Their Plates, New Survey Finds," http://www.aicr.org.

American Institute for Cancer Research. "New Survey Shows Americans Ignore Importance of Portion Size in Managing Weight," http://www.aicr.org.

Burros, M. "Losing Count of Calories as Plates Fill Up." *New York Times,* April 2, 1997, C: 1, 4.

DiDomenico, P. "Portion Size: How Much Is Too Much?" *Restaurants USA* 14 (1994): 18–21.

Fabricant, F. "From Mega-Food, Mega-Girth." *New York Times,* October 19, 1994, C: 1, 8.

Flegal, K. M., M. D. Carroll, and C. L. Johnson. "Prevalence and Trends in Obesity among U.S. Adults, 1999–2000." *Journal of the American Medical Association* 288 (2002): 1723–1727.

Flegal, K. M., M. D. Carroll, R. J. Kuczmarski, and C. L. Johnson. "Overweight and Obesity in the United States: Prevalence and Trends, 1960–1994." *International Journal of Obesity* 22 (1998): 39–47.

Food and Drug Administration. "FDA Proposes Action Plan to Confront Nation's Obesity Problem," http://www.fda.gov/default.htm.

Food and Nutrition Board, Institute of Medicine of the National Academy of Sciences. *Dietary Reference Intakes (DRI).* Washington, DC: National Academy of Sciences, 2002.

Goode, E. "The Gorge-Yourself Environment." *New York Times,* July 22, 2003: F1, 7.

Heimbach, J. T., A. S. Levy, and R. E. Schucker. "Declared Serving Sizes of Packaged Foods, 1977–86." *Food Technology* 44, no. 6 (1990): 82–90.

Hellmich, N. "Larger Portions Bring Larger Appetites." *USA Today,* January 22, 2003.

Jacobson, M. F., J. G. Hurley, and the Center for Science in the Public Interest. *Restaurant Confidential.* New York: Workman Publishing, 2002.

National Alliance for Nutrition and Activity. *From Wallet to Waistline: The Hidden Cost of Super Sizing.* Washington, DC: National Alliance for Nutrition and Activity, 2002.

National Center for Health Statistics, Centers for Disease Control. "Trends in Intake of Energy and Macronutrients—United States, 1971–2000." *Morbidity and Mortality Weekly Report* 53, no. 4 (2004): 80–82.

Nestle, M. *Food Politics: How the Food Industry Influences Nutrition and Health.* Berkeley: University of California Press, 2002.

Nielsen, S. J., and B. M. Popkin. "Patterns and Trends in Food Portion Sizes, 1977–1998." *Journal of the American Medical Association* 289 (2003): 450–453.

Ogden, C.L., C.D. Fryar, M.D. Carroll, K.M. Flegal. "Mean Body Weight, Height, and Body Mass Index, United States 1960–2002." Advance Data from Vital and Health Statistics, no. 347. Hyattsville, MD: National Center for Health Statistics, 2004.

Painter, J. E., B. Wansink, and J. B. Hieggelke. "How Visibility and Convenience Influence Candy Consumption." *Appetite* 38 (2002): 237–238.

Parker-Pope, T. "Eating for Six? Pasta Primavera Has Far More 'Servings' Than You Think." *Wall Street Journal,* May 20, 2003.

Putnam, J., J. Allshouse, and L. S. Kantor. "U.S. Per Capita Food Supply Trends: More Calories, Refined Carbohydrates, and Fats." *Food Review* 25 (2002): 2–15.

Rathje, W., and C. Murphy. *Rubbish! The Archaeology of Garbage.* New York: Harper-Collins, 1992.

Rolls, B. J. "The Supersizing of America: Portion Size and the Obesity Epidemic." *Nutrition Today* 38 (2003): 42–53.

Rolls, B. J., E. A. Bell, and B. A. Waugh. "Increasing the Volume of a Food by Incorporating Air Affects Satiety in Men." *American Journal of Clinical Nutrition* 72 (2000): 361–368.

Rolls, B. J., D. Engell, and L. L. Birch. "Serving Portion Size Influences 5-Year-Old But Not 3-Year-Old Children's Food Intakes." *Journal of the American Dietetic Association* 100 (2000): 232–234.

Rolls, B. J., E. L. Morris, and L. S. Roe. "Portion Size of Food Affects Energy Intake in Normal-Weight and Overweight Men and Women." *American Journal of Clinical Nutrition* 76 (2002): 1207–1213.

Rolls, B. J., L. S. Roe, and J. Meengs. "Salad and Satiety: Energy Density and Portion Size of a First-Course Salad Affect Energy Intake at Lunch." *Journal of the American Dietetic Association* 104 (2004): 1570–1576.

Rolls, B. J., L. S. Roe, T. V. E. Kral, J. S. Meengs, and D. E. Wall. "Increasing the Portion Size of a Packaged Snack Increases Energy Intake in Men and Women." *Appetite* 42 (2004): 63–69.

Rozin, P., K. Kabnick, E. Pete, C. Fischler, and C. Shields. "The Ecology of Eating: Smaller Portion Sizes in France than in the United States Help Explain the French Paradox." *Psychological Science* 14 (2003): 450–454.

Siegel, P. "The Completion Compulsion in Human Eating." *Psychological Reports* 3 (1957): 15–16.

Smiciklas-Wright, H., D. C. Mitchell, S. J. Mickle, J. D. Goldman, and A. Cook. "Food Commonly Eaten in the United States, 1989–1991 and 1994–1996: Are the Portion Sizes Changing?" *Journal of the American Dietetic Association* 103 (2003): 41–47.

U.S. Department of Agriculture. *The Food Guide Pyramid (Revised Edition).* Home and Garden Bulletin 252. Washington, DC: U.S. Department of Agriculture, 1996.

U.S. Department of Agriculture. *How Much Are You Eating?* Home and Garden Bulletin no. 267-1. Washington, DC: Center for Nutrition Policy and Promotion, 2002.

U.S. Department of Agriculture. *USDA Nutrient Database for Standard Reference.* Agricultural Research Service, Nutrient Data Laboratory home page, http://www.nal.usda.gov/fnic/foodcomp/.

U.S. Department of Health and Human Services, U.S. Department of Agriculture. *Di-*

etary Guidelines for Americans, 2005. 6th edition, Washington, DC: U.S. Government Printing Office, January 2005. http://www.healthierus.gov/dietaryguidelines.

Wansink, B. "Can Package Size Accelerate Usage Volume?" *Journal of Marketing* 60 (1996): 1–13.

Wansink, B., J. M. Painter, and J. North. "Why Visual Cues of Portion Size May Influence Intake." *Obesity Research* (March 2005), in press.

Wansink, B. "Study Reveals Package Size Can Accelerate Usage Volume." *Packaging Technology and Engineering* (February 1997): 42–45, 60.

Wansink, B., and L. R. Lindner. "Interaction between Forms of Fat Consumption and Restaurant Bread Consumption." *International Journal of Obesity* 27 (2003): 866–969.

Wansink, B., and S. B. Park. "At the Movies: How External Cues and Perceived Taste Impact Consumption Volume." *Food Quality and Preference* 12 (2001): 69–74.

Wansink, B., and K. Van Ittersum. "Bottoms Up! The Influence of Elongation on Pouring and Consumption Volume." *Journal of Consumer Research* 30 (2003): 455–463.

Young, L. R. *"Portion Sizes in the American Food Supply: Issues and Implications."* PhD dissertation, New York University, 2000.

Young, L. R. "Calorie Cop: How Fattening Is Mall Food?" *Your Diet* (Fall 2004): 24–25.

Young, L. R., and M. Nestle. "The Contribution of Expanding Portion Sizes to the U.S. Obesity Epidemic." *American Journal of Public Health* 92 (2002): 246–249.

Young, L. R., and M. Nestle. "Expanding Portion Sizes in the U.S. Marketplace: Implications for Nutrition Counseling." *Journal of the American Dietetic Association* 103 (2003): 231–234.

Young, L. R., and M. Nestle. "Food Labels Consistently Underestimate the Actual Weights of Single-Serving Baked Products." *Journal of the American Dietetic Association* 95 (1995): 1150–1151.

Young, L. R., and M. Nestle. "Portion Sizes in Dietary Assessment: Issues and Policy Implications." *Nutrition Reviews* 53 (1995): 149–158.

Young, L. R., and M. Nestle. "Variation in Perceptions of a 'Medium' Food Portion: Implications for Dietary Guidance." *Journal of the American Dietetic Association* 98 (1998): 458–459.

The following organizations, government agencies, and newsletters provide useful information on diet, nutrition, and health.

PROFESSIONAL ORGANIZATIONS AND CONSUMER GROUPS

American Academy of Pediatrics
141 Northwest Point Boulevard
Elk Grove Village, IL 60007–1098
(847) 434–4000
www.aap.org

American Cancer Society
1599 Clifton Road NE
Atlanta, GA 30329–4251
(800) ACS–2345
www.cancer.org

American Diabetes Association
1701 North Beauregard Street
Alexandria, VA 22311
(800) 342–2382
www.diabetes.org

American Dietetic Association
120 South Riverside Plaza, Suite 2000
Chicago, IL 60606–6995
(800) 877–1600 or (312) 899–0040
www.eatright.org

American Heart Association
Box BHG, National Center
7272 Greenville Avenue
Dallas, TX 75231
(800) AHA–USA1
www.americanheart.org

American Institute for Cancer Research
1759 R Street NW
Washington, DC 20009
(800) 843–8114 or (202) 328–7744
www.aicr.org

American Obesity Association
1250 24 Street NW, Suite 300
Washington, DC 20037
(800) 98–OBESE or (800) 986–2373
www.obesity.org

American Public Health Association
800 I Street NW
Washington, DC 20001–3710
(202) 777–2742
www.apha.org

Center for Science in the Public Interest
1875 Connecticut Avenue NW, Suite 300
Washington, DC 20009–5728
(202) 332–9110
www.cspinet.org

Consumers Union
101 Truman Avenue
Yonkers, NY 10703–1057
(914) 378–2000
www.consumersunion.org

International Food Information Council
Foundation
1100 Connecticut Avenue NW, Suite 430
Washington, DC 20036
(202) 296–6540
www.ific.org

Shape Up America!
N 4005 County Road U
Portage, WI 53901
(608) 742–1574
www.shapeup.org

GOVERNMENT AGENCIES

Centers for Disease Control and
Prevention
1600 Clifton Road NE
Atlanta, GA 30333
(404) 639–3311
www.cdc.gov

Food and Drug Administration
Office of Consumer Affairs, HFE 1
Room 16–85
5600 Fishers Lane
Rockville, MD 20857
(301) 443–1726
www.fda.gov

Food and Nutrition Information Center
National Agricultural Library, Room 304
10301 Baltimore Avenue
Beltsville, MD 20705–2351
(301) 504–5719
www.nal.usda.gov/fnic

National Academy of Sciences/National
Research Council
2101 Constitution Avenue NW
Washington, DC 20418
(202) 334–2000
www.nas.edu

National Heart, Lung, and Blood
Institute Health Information Center
PO Box 30105
Bethesda, MD 20824–0105
(301) 592–8573
www.nhlbi.nih.gov

National Institute of Diabetes and
Digestive Diseases Weight-Control
Information Network
1 WIN Way
Bethesda, MD 20892–3665
(877) 946–4627
www.niddk.nih.gov/health/nutrit/win.htm

National Institutes of Health
9000 Rockville Pike
Bethesda, MD 20892
(301) 496–2433
www.nih.gov

U.S. Department of Agriculture
14th Street and Independence Avenue SW
Washington, DC 20250
(202) 720–2791
www.fns.usda.gov/fncs

USDA Center for Nutrition Policy and Promotion
1120 20th Street NW, Suite 200
North Lobby
Washington, DC 20036
(800) 687–2258 or (202) 418–2312
www.cnpp.usda.gov

U.S. Department of Health and Human Services
200 Independence Avenue SW
Washington, DC 20201
(202) 619–0257
www.os.dhhs.gov

World Health Organization
Regional Office
525 23rd Street NW
Washington, DC 20037
(202) 974–3000
www.who.org

NUTRITION AND HEALTH NEWSLETTERS

University of California, Berkeley Wellness Letter
School of Public Health
PO Box 420148
Palm Coast, FL 32142
(800) 829–9170
www.berkeleywellness.com

Consumer Reports on Health
A Publication of Consumers Union
PO Box 5385
Harlan, IA 51593
(914) 378–2000
www.ConsumerReports.org/health

Environmental Nutrition
PO Box 420235
Palm Coast, FL 32142
(800) 829–5384
www.environmentalnutrition.com

Nutrition Action Health Letter
Center for Science in the Public Interest
1875 Connecticut Avenue NW, Suite 300
Washington, DC 20009–5728
(202) 332–9110
www.cspinet.org

Tufts University Health and Nutrition Letter
The Friedman School of Nutrition Science and Policy
PO Box 420235
Palm Coast, FL 32142
(800) 274–7581
www.healthletter.tufts.edu

WEIGHT-LOSS PROGRAMS/GROUPS

Overeaters Anonymous
World Service Office
PO Box 44021
Rio Rancho, NM 87124
(505) 891–2664
www.oa.org

Weight Watchers International, Inc.
Consumer Affairs Department/IN
175 Crossways Park West
Woodbury, NY 11797
(800) 651–6000
www.weightwatchers.com

TOPS (Take Off Pounds Sensibly)
4575 South Fifth Street
PO Box 07360
Milwaukee, WI 53207–0360
(800) 932–8677 or (414) 482–4620
www.tops.org

RESIDENTIAL WEIGHT-LOSS CENTERS

Duke University Diet and Fitness Center
804 West Trinity Avenue
Durham, NC 27701
(800) 362–8446
www.dukedietcenter.org

Pritikin Longevity Center and Spa
19735 Turnberry Way
Aventura, FL 33180
(800) 327–4914
www.pritikin.com

Green Mountain at Fox Run
Box 164, Fox Lane
Ludlow, VT 05149
(800) 448–8106
www.fitwoman.com

Structure House
3017 Pickett Road
Durham, NC 27705
(800) 553–0052
www.structurehouse.com

The Hilton Head Health Institute
14 Valencia Road, Box 7138
Hilton Head Island, SC 29938
(800) 292–2440
www.hhhealth.com